# PRAISE FOR *LIVING WELLNESS*

As a provider of healthcare for women, I encourage my patients to read *Living Wellness*. Specifically, the information on osteoporosis and its prevention is accurate, thorough, and insightful. *Living Wellness* is a "must-have" for one who seeks a lifestyle of health and wellness!

Dr. Daniel T. Chow, MD

I am pleased to see a holistic approach in *Living Wellness* that includes nutrition, wellness, exercise, and a faith-based foundation. Such a combination breathes fuel for the mind, body, and soul.

Kristine Haertl, PhD, OTR/L, FAOTA, author, professor

In a world that shifts like sand, *Living Wellness* is something to stand on. Ashley Darkenwald speaks to your body, mind, and soul. She speaks to wholeness and health. Open these pages and you will be inspired from head to toe to heart!

Bjorn Dixon, MDiv, pastor, the WHY Church in Elk River, Minnesota

I thoroughly enjoyed reading *Living Wellness*. I highly recommend it to those desiring to make a minor or major change in their wellness. *Living Wellness* is well-researched, balanced, simple to understand, and a great tool for individuals and families who are serious about improving their health.

Carole Joy Seid, MA in education,
speaker and consultant for home educators

Great book! *Living Wellness* will give you many ideas and great motivation to get healthy from the inside out. I am sure you will pick up several ideas from this book, even if you are a well-seasoned reader in the areas of health and weight loss. The ideas are attractively presented with pictures, charts, and graphs, making it easy and interesting to read. Read it and see if your health doesn't improve! Excellent work, Ashley Darkenwald.

Dr. Mark Virkler, President of Christian Leadership University

There are very few readings that will inspire, energize, and transform one's mindset like what Ashley Darkenwald has put together in *Living Wellness*. We all need inspiration and ways to reach heights that are often difficult to achieve. Ashley has designed a way to be successful for all walks of life. To the professional with time restraints and the person looking for consistent motivation—commit to reading *Living Wellness* a day or two every week and you will find a path of positive opportunities for a lifetime. This is a multiple, MUST-read journey!

Steve Fessler, PGA professional

Ashley not only taught me how to exercise properly, she taught me about nutrition and encouraged me to continue to push myself. After losing over 24 pounds and 6 inches off of my waist, I have kept the inches and pounds off, I am still wearing a size 0, and it has been almost three years! I have more energy to keep up with my three kids and I am healthier and stronger than ever. I have never looked or felt better!

Kari Dwinnell, age 44, *Living Wellness* testimonial

Reading *Living Wellness* and working with Ashley helps me stay focused on my goals and adapt them when my life circumstances change. When I gained over 50 pounds with my pregnancy, even though it was discouraging, I knew with InFIT Workouts and Ashley's help and support I would get back to my old self again! Her passion, commitment, knowledge, and sincere desire over the last five years have transformed my life, and I will forever be grateful!

Alissa Henriksen, age 31, co-president–CorTalent

The InFIT approach to fitness in *Living Wellness* is unique and so were my results. In a matter of months, I broke through my plateau, retooled my workouts, documented a road map to reach my goals, and then drove accountability to follow that plan. I just turned 42 years old and with Ashley Darkenwald's help, I did so in the best shape of my life.

Joseph Banack, *Living Wellness* testimonial

After living out the principles in *Living Wellness* for over five years, *I am in the best shape of my life*, physically, mentally, and emotionally. I feel as though the whole-health approach to wellness helped me achieve my 100-pound weight loss journey. I lost the weight 5 years ago, kept it off, and gained a new appreciation for life and health. With the guidance of Ashley and *Living Wellness*, I changed my life with small, consistent steps—and you can too!

Laura Lium, age 42, *Living Wellness* testimonial

Ashley Darkenwald and *Living Wellness* have transformed the way we think about food. Little by little, we have given up soda, reduced packaged foods, balanced our salt intake, and we make smarter choices when eating out. *Together we have lost over 100 pounds and I, Donna, am no longer pre-diabetic!* And we are not even on a diet. With the practical knowledge in *Living Wellness*, we enjoy living a healthy lifestyle. We have come to ask ourselves, "Is this food choice *Ashley approved?*" Together, we love living in the freedom that comes with exceptional health.

Donna and Chris Schwab, *Living Wellness* testimonial

**BECAUSE YOU WERE CREATED FOR MORE THAN MEDIOCRE**

# LIVING WELLNESS

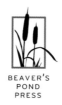

BEAVER'S
POND
PRESS

The *infit* Approach
to Proven Weight Loss
and Dynamic Nutrition

Ashley Darkenwald, BA, CPT, PES

Editor: Catherine Long
Proofreader: Leah Noel

ISBN 13: 978-1-59298-946-1

Library of Congress Catalog Number: 2013922718

Printed in the United States of America

First Printing: 2014

18  17  16  15  14     5  4  3  2  1

Cover and interior design by James Monroe Design, LLC.

Beaver's Pond Press, Inc.
7108 Ohms Lane
Edina, MN  55439-2129
(952) 829-8818

www.BeaversPondPress.com

To order, visit www.BeaversPondBooks.com
or call (800) 901-3480. Reseller discounts available.

# DEDICATION

**Mom, this book is for you.** You taught me to listen to myself among so many voices. I love you more than I can say in words. You loved me before I was born, you never gave up on me when I was down, and you poured into me even when I had nothing to give back. Thank you for giving me your strength and your courage. May God pour out blessings on you forever and ever.

# CONTENTS

# FOREWORD

You have picked up a very special book. A rare gem in a vast, gray landscape. Let me tell you about that landscape and this gem.

I am the pastor of a church that calls a large fitness center our home. Every day at the office I see people stream in and out the doors to attend a class, or run on a treadmill, or swim in the pool, or lift weights. I am also the husband of a personal trainer—a fitness professional and hobby triathlete. Every day I see her planning PT sessions, or reading the latest fitness magazines, or training for her next event. Fitness is of ever-increasing importance in our culture, especially as we battle back against the forces of obesity, diabetes, and heart disease—to name a few. There is a growing fitness movement across our communities and it is exciting to see!

But there is something much more subtle that has caught my eye. Of all the people pursuing greater fitness, some seem to attain something more—something deeper, something more life-changing than just a trimmer wasteline. Rather than just greater fitness, *some people find true health.*

Ashley Darkenwald knows about finding true health. She knows about the deeper, life-changing aspects of fitness. And in this book she will take you there.

*Living Wellness* is a gem in the vast landscape of fitness literature and quick-fix philosophies. The market is cluttered with approaches that address one aspect of health. There are an array of books on fitness, and some are effective in telling you what to do to lose weight. But many miss the why and how to get you there for the long haul. Ashley will take you from fitness to wellness, from nutrition to wholeness, and from health all the way to life!

The spiritual element of your health may or may not be something you have thought about very much. Wherever you are in your faith journey, *do not hesitate to read on.* This is not a Christian book dressed up in fitness lingo. This is a fitness book with a spiritual foundation. Nothing here is overspiritualized. And yet nothing is overlooked or dismissed. What you will find here is wholeness and balance.

This wholistic approach to *Living Wellness* reminds me of something . . . Jesus was once asked, "What is the greatest commandment?" Quoting words from the Old Testament, he answered, "Love the Lord your God with all your heart and with all your soul and with all your strength and with all your mind" (Luke 10:27). To love God might easily be considered just a soul issue, or maybe a heart issue. But Jesus also saw it as something to be done with all your strength and with all your mind. He blew the regular categories out of the water and saw you and I as whole people created in the image of God. What if we applied the same lesson to fitness and nutrition?

What if we invited the soul and the mind into this conversation about the body? *Living Wellness* has.

As profound as *Living Wellness* will be for you, it is remarkably straightforward and easy to grasp. In these pages you will find out why you need certain nutrients to be fit and healthy, and why others harm your body. You will see illustrated step-by-step workouts and stretching pages. And you will read about the honest need we all have for spiritual health.

In a world where we are bombarded with fast workouts and fad diets, this book shines. You have discovered a gem. Read it and live it. Be blessed!

Bjorn Dixon, MDiv, pastor of the WHY Church
in Elk River, Minnesota

# INTRODUCTION

Achieving your health goals on your own can be a frustrating experience. There are hundreds of diet plans, exercise programs, and weight loss drugs all promising everyone the same results. And still the large majority of people participating find themselves giving up and feeling worse than when they started. The fitness industry wants to sell you a "one-size-fits-all" program that fit *only a small number of people's needs*. That is why some are successful and why everyone else moves on to the next miracle program hoping it is the right fit. *You* are the reason why I created a new program that begins and ends with what *you*, as an individual, want to achieve. Not just in terms of fitness or nutrition or even motivation, but also for the whole human being wellness, which is what we all want but are hopeless to reach on our own. My name is Ashley Darkenwald. I have been working in the fitness arena for over a decade. I have seen the broken-promise fitness cycle repeat itself over and over. So let me introduce you to *Living Wellness*.

*Living Wellness* is functional, integrated, raw, and motivated. You need clear goals to achieve wellness, but what the world is discovering is that it is just as important to be part of a support structure that encourages one another to fight on and become our ideal selves. I encourage you to read *Living Wellness* with a small group or a close friend. If you decide to make this journey with others, your group will be your foundation. Friends come alongside you, celebrate your success, and pick you up if you stumble. Couple

this with proven instruction, and you have a comprehensive program that cannot fail. Even if you decide to follow the guide by yourself, you still have the perfect road map for success.

## Functional

The functional exercises in *Living Wellness* deliver strength from the inside out, making your *whole* body strong and less prone to everyday and chronic injury. Functional is not doing endless curls, leg presses, and bench presses. Yes, that makes us look better on the outside, but eventually even people with incredibly strong arms and legs will bend over to pick something up and throw their back out. InFIT workouts assist in your appearance and in your life.

## Integrated

*Living Wellness* integrates nutrition, fitness, mind, and soul, all functioning together to bring you *complete* health and wellness. Think about integrated nutrition. How many times have you set a fantastic meal plan for yourself that hopelessly unravels the second that you find yourself on the road, at a party, or starving while getting fuel? Rigid meal plans are great if you are the kind of person who can plan for every foreseeable interference or interruption in daily routine. For the rest of us, *we need a plan that can adapt and evolve with real life*. Our lives are never totally structured and serene.

## Raw

*Living Wellness* is raw. Raw is reality. Always having the time to cook, get to the gym, or motivate yourself in the morning is a utopia that the majority of us do not live in. Life is unpredictable, wild; it is raw. *Living Wellness* takes your reality and integrates it into your total wellness plan. Raw, optimal nutrition is choosing the most nourishing and the least genetically modified, processed, and packaged food. *Optimal nutrition is not about, "is this food good or bad." Optimal nutrition is about choosing your best option in the given circumstance.*

Raw fitness is doing InFIT Workouts that use your own body weight, gravity, and/or balance to strengthen your core muscles that are used every day, workouts for home *or* at the gym. Having a solid, adaptive workout and nutrition plan is important, but it all means nothing without a mind and spirit uncluttered by insecurity and fear, which develop when we are isolated. This is why we need motivation.

## Motivated

The secret weapon of *Living Wellness* is motivation. Lack of motivation is the number one killer of *lasting* health and fitness progress. Motivation in *Living Wellness* is similar to a tiny snowball; you need to make the decision to change your lifestyle, to be honest and transparent with your support network, and to start the ball rolling with your thoughts and actions. After that, the momentum, efficient and effective workouts, accountability, meal ideas, affirmations, and the proven information in *Living Wellness* will turn your small snowball of motivation into an avalanche force toward your goals and a healthier you.

## InFIT

*So much is missing from the traditional path of fitness.* Think about finding your way around in a foreign country, trying to understand road signs. The signs are simply not created for you. This is how many people describe navigating through the plethora of available health and weight loss information. *Living Wellness* is the guide who comes alongside you, translating the vast amounts of information available into the path that makes sense and gets you to where you, specifically, want to go. If you are ready to start journeying on your wellness path, if you are ready to get healthy, then join the others, like you, and get ready to get InFIT!

# HOW TO USE THIS BOOK

*Living Wellness* is your complete reference guide for nutrition education, proven weight loss information, and life-changing health and fitness answers. As a home educator, I use *Living Wellness* and the InFIT approach with my children as a well-being and spiritual education course by reading through the material, praying through the affirmations, preparing the healthy meals, and even practicing the workouts together as a family. Depending on your goals, you may not need to read *Living Wellness* from cover to cover. Write in this book with a pencil so that when you read through a second or a third time, you can update your responses with your new perspective on health and wellness. My prayer is that you will find nourishment, education, and encouragement, however you choose to read through *Living Wellness*.

*For improved, long-term health and wellness*: Look at the table of contents. First read the chapters that speak to your body's individual needs. Read your selected chapters carefully, highlighting sections that may need review. Be sure to practice the workouts *in order*. They are conveniently designed in 20-minute (1 set), 40-minute, or 60-minute sessions, depending on how many sets you perform. Each workout adds complexity from the previous workout, building a strong, cumulative physical foundation. Finally, remember to foam roll and stretch your muscles daily using the illustrated stretches in this book.

*For weight loss*: Read the first three chapters. These chapters lay the foundation of science and math, not just educating you on *what* to do, but on *how* and *why* weight loss is important. Once you know *how* to lose weight, move on to the subjects that you struggle with on your weight loss journey. For example, if you do not like the taste of most vegetables, read "Eat a Rainbow for Weight Loss." If you are ever constipated, read "Full of Fiber: Constipation Cures." Do not neglect any single chapter, but feel free to maneuver around. Each chapter teaches you how to balance your body's macro and micro nutrient needs, making weight loss efforts *easier* than without the education. Be sure to practice the workouts *in order*. They are conveniently designed in 20-minute (1 set), 40-minute, or 60-minute sessions, depending on how many sets you perform. Each workout adds complexity from the previous workout, building a strong, cumulative physical foundation. Consistent exercise builds strength and burns calories, two must-have components for weight loss. Finally, remember to foam roll and stretch your muscles daily using the illustrated stretches in this book.

*For spiritual well-being*: Read the affirmation sections. Take your time thinking through each affirmation, individually or with a friend. Meditate on the scripture verses, answer the questions, and reflect on the affirmations in prayer. Take time each day to practice the stretching and foam rolling exercises while performing deep breathing. Stretching and deep breathing promote relaxation, stress reduction, and spiritual well-being.

*For small group study*: First read a section of the book as individuals. Then get together as a group, on a weekly or bimonthly basis, to talk through the information. Discuss your thoughts on the S2L (Share 2 Learn) and practice sections. Listen to each person's challenges and offer encouragement as to what worked well. Practice the workouts and stretching sections individually and as a group. In a group setting, reading *Living Wellness* is a powerful motivator to keep you on track with your goals and strengthen your relationships with others.

## Overview of *Living Wellness*

### Chapter Material

Most individuals know *what* to do to lose weight and get in shape. Eat less and exercise more, right? If it were only that easy, we would all be incredibly thin and healthy. The *Living Wellness* chapter material is designed to teach you *why* we should make certain choices: Why do you need protein and healthy dietary fat? What do vegetables have to do with weight loss? What is the correct ratio of Omega-3s and Omega-6s and why does your brain health depend on that balance? Over a decade of personal training and nutrition coaching, and being the owner and operator of several fitness businesses, have given me the insight into *what you want to know and what works*. I learned that if we know *why* something works, we are significantly more inclined to make lasting change and positive habits a permanent part of our lives. *Living Wellness* answers your questions in a clear, easy-to-follow guidebook, giving you the knowledge and motivation to make informed decisions about your health and wellness.

### InFIT Workouts

The workouts in this book are designed using the proven and effective Optimum Performance Training™ (OPT) model from the National Academy of Sports Medicine. Working first through stabilization, strength, and then power, your body will be less likely to get injured and more likely to become strong and healthy. Read the introduction "Getting Fit" in Chapter 1 before you begin the workouts: You will learn how much weight to use and how many repetitions to perform. Be sure to check with your physician before beginning a new workout routine.

### Road Map to Success

Track your progress and measure your success. You do not need to fill out every matrix in the Road Map to Success section to make the effort worth your time. But some health tracking is always better than none. Look at each category of goals and determine the most important objectives for you. Start by filling out the "Goal" and "Actual" sections until they become habit. For example, if you are not drinking the recommended amount of water per day, write down your goal in Road Map to Success. Track how much water you are drinking per day until you have consistently met your objective for several weeks. Once you have created a habit, you no longer need to track it. Habits may come and go. Pay attention to your body and your nutritional needs. You may need to track certain goals more closely in various seasons of your life.

### Living Affirmations

My renewed spirituality after high school fueled my passion for health and wellness. God *personally* calls each one of us to be healthy. *Living Wellness* is meant to be a guide for your mind, body, and soul. I write to educate and inspire you toward a healthier mind and body. But health does not end there. Fellow colleague and friend Christina Zaczkowski, MA theology and education, CPT, joins us on our journey with chapter by chapter affirmations that will challenge and nourish your soul. Immigrating to America from Germany in 2010, to the industry of health and fitness as a personal trainer and educator, Christina has a unique perspective on faith and fitness and their absolute connectedness.

I meditated on whether to include a spiritual component to this book because it risks alienating readers. Yet, the answer was clear when a mentor inquired how my soul affects fitness and how fitness affects my soul. Both are absolutely connected. I cannot separate spirituality from my health. I must deliver my message completely and truthfully, with the whole person in focus. This book is written from a Christian perspective. This is not meant to convert or offend anyone. *Living Wellness* is meant to be a guidebook to better health. Jump to the chapters that speak to your needs, or read the whole book cover to cover. Complete health includes your mind, body, and soul, and I encourage you to read *Living Wellness* wherever you are in your faith walk. I am humbled as I share my health discoveries with you.

**Use this key when practicing workouts:**

# KEY:

Alternate = **ALT**

Dumbbell = **DB**

Isometric = **ISO**

Medicine Ball = **MB**

Stability Ball = **SB**

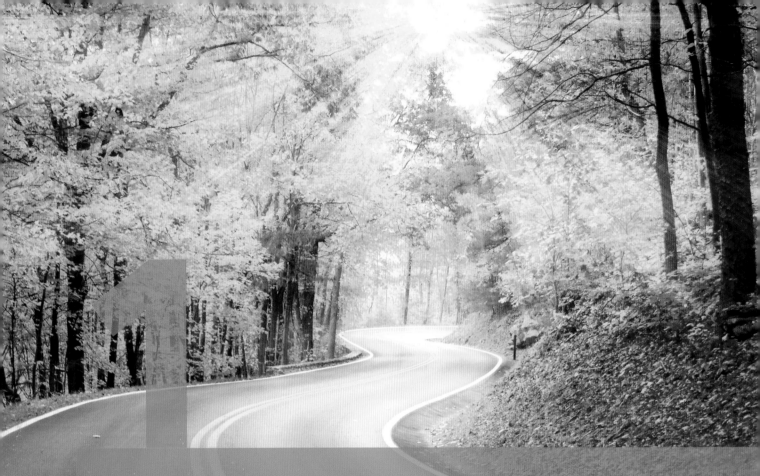

# PREPARING YOUR
# ROAD MAP TO SUCCESS

## Principle Thoughts:

1. What is health?

2. Are you healthy?

3. What are your nutrition goals?

4. What are your fitness goals?

5. How do you start your new plan?

I have not always been fit and healthy. In high school, I decided to change course from a three-season athlete to a theater performer. This dramatically reduced my activity level, and I gained weight. If you had asked my friends, they would not have classified me as overweight, but you could imagine the surprise when I lost 20 pounds in college from a consistent running routine! I did not start out running miles and miles per day. I made a commitment to get to the gym every day for at least three minutes. Yes, just three minutes. I heard a motivational speaker say that anyone can make time for three minutes per day for something important. I was working full time to pay for college and taking a substantial course load to graduate early.

Three minutes per day of exercise for one semester: This simple commitment developed into a habit and a discipline for physical fitness that led to my unforeseen weight loss, rejuvenated interest in health, and passion for helping others find their start to a lifelong journey of health and whole-person wellness.

Looking back at those three minutes per day, it seemed unusual that I did not strive for more or make it a goal to run marathons like some of my friends. I was young and able, but also tired and unhealthy. The important part was that I made consistent, daily decisions to put my health first and continue to practice healthy habits even when I did not feel like it. I learned that I could not make the decision to "become healthy" and then walk away. There were hurdles and setbacks, injuries and broken dreams—I had to make a decision with every new challenge: Would I return to health? Oftentimes I was a slow learner. Looking back at my journey, I cannot even believe what I thought was healthy ten years ago!

I know that if you do not grow up learning healthy habits, adults have a hard time changing them. If that is you today or you did learn healthy habits but fell away when you landed a career or started having kids, *my encouragement for you is strong*. I have seen thousands of lives transformed with the daily decision to put health first. I was able to learn healthy habits after a lifetime of *un*health, I lost weight when I never thought I needed to, and I continue to learn every day that health is a worthwhile journey. I am not alone. Your enjoyment of health will increase with practice. Eventually, you will watch people around you transform as they catch the contagious health bug. Let me help you catch your health bug.

> *"People by and large become what they think about themselves."*
> —BOB ROTELLA

Do you want to improve your health?

☐ Yes  ☐ No  ☐ Maybe

Why?

Nutrition Goal Examples:

Eat one to two more servings of produce per day.

Drink twenty more ounces of water per day.

Avoid processed and packaged foods.

Pack meals and snacks for an afternoon or evening out rather than relying solely on fast food.

*What you put in your body affects how you feel.*

How do you feel about yourself and your body?

## Welcome to Health!

Imagine hopping in a new car, spending money on fuel, buying supplies for your trip, throwing your nicest clothes in a suitcase, and then setting out on a road trip adventure. If you have endless resources and no responsibilities, you may have a great time driving aimlessly around the state or even the country. But at the end of your trip, would you call it a success? Would you have spent your most valuable resource, your time, wisely based on where you wanted to go and what you wanted to see? What if you encountered turbulent weather or a flat tire? Would you be able to flexibly change your course without a plan? If you do not have a road map, goals, and a plan, you probably wasted your time, energy, and money.

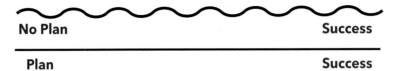

| No Plan | Success |
| Plan | Success |

*You do not have to keep driving your health with no plan.* Change course! Slow down with me for a season of reflection and education. Assess the state of your health, where you want to go, how you want to feel when you wake up, and what you will experience with your friends and family with your new vitality. Let us finally begin the journey to be the person you have always wanted to be, starting with the end (your success) in mind.

> *After a great workout, I am the happiest person in the world.*
>
> Kristie S.
> InFIT instructor

The more clearly you see yourself right now, the more clearly you will see where you want to make changes in your lifestyle.

> *"To be physically healthy, people will realize that they must take care of their inner being. To be healthy within, people will realize that they must take care of their physical body."*
>
> Harold Eberle

Assessing your current physical, emotional, and spiritual environment, and preparing a road map for success are the most important objectives for life-changing results. The idea of knowing oneself is quoted by scholars and philosophers throughout history. To know yourself better, take your time filling out this assessment, frequently used at my fitness studio, InFIT. Ask yourself, *What is health?* and *Am I healthy?* The most important journey of your life depends on it.

## InFIT Assessment

### Nutrition

What are your short-term (one to six months) nutrition goals?

_____

_____

What are your long-term (six months to one year) nutrition goals?

_____

_____

Why do you want to improve your nutrition?

_____

What has kept you from achieving your nutrition goals? Be specific.

_____

Why?

_____

Please describe everything you ate and drank yesterday with approximate calories (if known):

| Food | Calories |
|------|----------|
| Breakfast: | |
| Snacks: | |
| Lunch: | |
| Snacks: | |
| Dinner: | |
| Snacks: | |
| Beverages: | |
| Based on yesterday's account, approximately how many calories are you eating per day? | |

Describe any diets you have tried in the past:

_____

If you have dieted in the past, are you still experiencing success?

_____

Have you ever kept a wellness or food/exercise journal? _____

**Trainer's Recommendation:** I highly recommend keeping a wellness journal! See below for an example if you plan to keep a wellness journal.

| Time | Nutrition | Calories | Exercise | Water | Feel | Sleep |
|------|-----------|----------|----------|-------|------|-------|
| 7 am | 1/2 cup yogurt 1/4 cup berries | 180 total | 1 hour bike ride | 20 ounces | Great today! | 8 hours |

## Keep a Wellness Journal

*There is one strong recommendation from this book, and it is to keep a detailed wellness journal*, even for a short period of time. You will learn crucial information about yourself and your eating and exercise habits. Even if you have kept a journal in the past, please try again. You are a different person now.

There are other ways to keep a wellness journal that are technical and computer friendly like using a fitness application (app) on your

Use this area as a scratch pad for math calculations.

Are you going to start tracking your calories in a notebook, on a computer, or with a mobile application?

Yes/No

Why?

What could get in the way of tracking your calories consistently (e.g., time, motivation, difficulty)?

How can you overcome these challenges?

Use this area as a scratch pad for math calculations.

Is this math frustrating you? If so, I understand.

Talk it through with someone. Even if you are not going to commit to counting calories, you should have a basic understanding of how many your body needs so that when you reach for a 600-calorie muffin at the coffee shop, you *stop* and think about how that *one* muffin might be *half of your daily calorie needs. If you know how much energy your body needs, you will be able to make wiser decisions.*

smart phone or a calorie and exercise tracking website. Finding the one that is right for you is important for long-term success. If you try one that is not the right fit, keep looking. There are so many to choose from. Ask around and find the right one for you!

Before we look at the science behind managing your weight, let us pause for a moment and reflect on the importance of the following equation. You are about to calculate how many calories you need to maintain your body weight and how many calories you need to decrease body fat. *If your goal is to lose weight and you do nothing else in this book but track calories and stay at your weight-loss calorie goal (and you have no metabolic disorders), you will lose weight.* So can we all just follow this formula and lose weight? No more diets, no more pills, no more clueless hours at the gym . . .

## The Science Behind Managing Your Weight

The following formula is science and math, and it works. However, the key to balancing a healthy lifestyle without starving or spending clueless hours at the gym is also knowing the *right combination of foods and practicing functional, efficient fitness.* Read on.

### Calculating Your Success

1. Calculate your basal metabolic rate (BMR). Your BMR is the amount of energy your body burns doing basic functions such as breathing and circulating blood. Do the equation in the appropriate formula from left to right. See below for examples.

*If you are under age thirty, do this equation:*

(0.0621 x your weight/2.2 + 2.0357) x 240 = BMR (multiply by 1.05 for men)

(0.0621 x _____ /2.2 + 2.0357) x 240 = _____ (BMR)

*If you are over age thirty, do this equation:*

(0.0342 x your weight/2.2 + 3.5377) x 240 = BMR (multiply by 1.05 for men)

(0.0342 x _____ /2.2 + 3.5377) x 240 = _____ (BMR)

2. Find your average daily activity level. Do not count exercise:

a. You have a sedentary lifestyle (i.e., driving or desk job): *Factor: 1.1*

b. Lightly active (i.e., nurse or teacher): *Factor: 1.2*

c. Heavily active (i.e., server or construction): *Factor: 1.3*

3. Multiply your BMR and your activity level (factor). This is your approximate number of calories for maintenance: _____

> This total is your approximate daily calorie requirement. To maintain your body weight, stick as closely as you can to that number.

### Female Example

Let us look at an example of a BMR equation for a forty-five-year-old female who weighs 180 pounds.

1. (0.0342 x 180/2.2 + 3.5377) x 240 = 1,520

2. Sedentary lifestyle = 1.1 factor

3. 1,520 x 1.1 = 1,672 is the approximate number of her maintenance calories.

### Male Example

Let us look at an example of a BMR equation for a forty-five-year-old male who weighs 200 pounds.

1. (0.0342 x 200/2.2 + 3.5377) x 240 x 1.05 = 1,751

2. Lightly active = 1.2 factor

3. 1,751 x 1.2 = 2,101 is the approximate number of his maintenance calories.

Maintenance calories indicate that if you eat that amount of calories per day without exercising, you will not gain or lose weight. *You will maintain your current body weight.*

## How Do You Decrease Body Fat?

To decrease body fat, we need a calorie deficit. We must consume less than what we need and/or burn more calories than we consume with daily activity and exercise.

A 3,500-calorie surplus or deficit equals 1 pound of body fat gained or lost, respectively.

For a weight loss goal of 1 pound per week, subtract *500 calories* from your daily *maintenance* calories.

Approximate daily weight loss calorie goal: _____

Again, it is my strongest recommendation that you keep a wellness journal. While some programs suggest that no calorie counting is needed to lose weight, those plans are usually so strict that most people cannot adhere to them long-term. And because most people have a limited understanding of calories, they end

**What is Health?**

There are hundreds of different definitions of health. Don Colbert, MD, offers a wonderful definition using the following seven pillars to asses health:

1. Water

2. Sleep and rest

3. Living foods

4. Exercise

5. Detoxification

6. Nutritional supplements

7. Coping with stress

Which one(s) do you need to improve?

I have never met one person who is 100% happy with his or her body. Let us love and honor our bodies the way they are right now and watch our exteriors transform out of love, rather than self-hatred.

up failing the program. Calories are the very unit of energy for all foods and beverages. We do not need to (and we should not) obsess over calories to have a solid understanding of how many we need and how many calories are in our foods and beverages. Once we know our bodies, our cravings, and what our bodies need, *we will no longer need to keep track of calories, water, exercise, and how we feel on a regular basis!* One health goal is to learn your body's needs so you can respond when your body speaks to you.

**Weekly Review**

Review this chapter often; once a week would be optimal in the beginning. Remember, everyone's definition of health varies. Some people think health is a number on a scale, some people think it is how you feel, some people think it is the habits you create and maintain. Good health is a combination of all these. The World Health Organization (WHO) states:

- Health is a state of complete physical, mental, and social well-being and not merely the absence of disease or infirmity

*Are you going to keep a journal now?*

I will not judge either way. I will tell you that I have been in the industry long enough to know that the clients who have lasting results in weight management use a wellness journal (even for a short period of time).

Summing up this section in your own words, how do you decrease body fat?

_____

(If you said something like *burn more or consume less calories than you need,* you are correct.)

## What Are Calories?

A calorie is a unit of heat energy measured in all foods and beverages. There are dozens of programs that try to simplify counting calories: points, net carbs, fat grams, sugar alcohol, servings, et cetera. However, these programs are missing one of the main ingredients in weight loss, calories! When we understand what calories are and how they function in our bodies, we can take charge of our weight and our bodies' needs.

In the same breath, I was recently reminded of a client who sees significantly more success when she does not micro-manage her calories, but instead participates in training or group fitness classes held at my studio, InFIT. With the help of friends and professionals, my client daily puts nutrition and fitness in the front of her mind. She has lost weight without counting calories. In my experience, she is among the minority of people. However, if you experience more success managing your weight without counting calories, be sure to take that approach. *You know what is best for your body!*

Remember, there is no one-size-fits-all approach to effective weight management. Give one method a try, and if you are not satisfied with the result, try again with a different approach!

## Continuing the InFIT Assessment—Are You Healthy?

How many servings of fruits and veggies do you consume per day? Keep track for three days and record it here:

Day 1 _____ servings

Day 2 _____ servings

Day 3 _____ servings

**Trainer's Recommendation:** You should consume at least five to seven servings of produce per day.

If you are not consuming at least five to seven servings of fruits and veggies per day, making this small change will have a significant impact *instantly* on your health and your weight. We will cover this amazing secret in more detail in Chapter 5, but for now, we cannot wait that long. Fruits and vegetables offer vitamins, minerals, anti-oxidants, fiber, water, and they reduce the risk of disease, diabetes, and high blood pressure. Fruits and veggies also help you feel full without excessive calories. You can eat a whole plate of vegetables for about 150 calories. A whole plate of french fries equal about *1,000* calories! Eat vegetables even if you do not love them; your pallet will change.

Next, do you take supplements? _____

**Trainer's Recommendation:** For most individuals, supplementation is recommended. See Chapter 11 for more details.

How much water do you drink per day? Keep track for three days and record it here:

Day 1 _____ ounces

Day 2 _____ ounces

Day 3 _____ ounces

**Trainer's Recommendation:** You should consume half your ideal body weight in ounces of water per day.

How much do you weigh? _____

How much water should you be drinking per day? _____ ounces

Your body is made up of approximately 60% water. Water is responsible for bringing nutrients into and removing waste from every cell in your body. Water also aids in digestion, balances body fluids, helps you feel full, keeps your muscles energized, keeps your skin elastic, and flushes your kidneys and liver. After consuming enough fruits and vegetables, drinking the appropriate amount of water every day will have a profound impact on how you look and feel.

**Tip from Your Trainer:** Keep a reusable (glass) bottle nearby and fill it often!

**Fitness Goal Examples:**

- Start walking three minutes per day.
- Join a fitness center with a friend.
- Practice strength training at least once a week.
- Stretch your muscles every day.
- Change your current fitness routine.

*Find something you enjoy! Exercise should not be viewed as a form of punishment, but a way to make you feel better!*

AMY P.
INFIT INSTRUCTOR

**Water Note**

Take into consideration water needs and obesity. The recommendation of half your body weight in ounces per day of water is based on your healthy goal weight.

## Make a Plan for Overcoming Health and Fitness Excuses

She talks to each of us in different ways. What is the Excuse Muse whispering in your ear? Circle all that apply:

• I am too busy • Temptation is too strong • I am afraid I will fail • I am just too tired • I am not motivated • Bad habits are more fun • I am distracted • I am not worth the hassle • I want to get back at someone with my bad choices • My spouse is not worth the work it takes for me to look good • If I lose weight, people who have been nagging me to lose weight will have won

What is your daily plan to practice overcoming the Excuse Muse?

_____

Who can you discuss your nutrition goals with?

_____

Do you have any additional nutrition thoughts? Remember, the more clear your road map is, the more success you will have getting to your destination.

_____

## Physical Fitness

What are your short-term (zero to six months) fitness goals?

_____

What are your long-term (six months to one year) fitness goals?

_____

Why do you want to improve your fitness?

_____

What has kept you from achieving your goals?

_____

Please describe your current exercise routine (this will help you determine your intensity level as you begin the InFIT Workouts and Cardio Plan):

_____

How many days per week are you doing cardio exercise: _____

**Trainer's Recommendation:** Adding three to five times (thirty to sixty minutes each) of cardio per week improves your weight and heart health.

How many days per week are you doing strength training: _____

**Trainer's Recommendation:** Adding one to three times (twenty to sixty minutes each) of strength training per week improves your muscle tone and body composition.

Have you ever followed a structured exercise program? _____

If so, what was your experience?

_____

What is your plan to incorporate more movement into your schedule?

_____

## Getting Fit!

This is exciting! You are about to begin a workout program that is proven, effective, and full of illustrations to ensure safety and accuracy. Remember, you should always obtain permission from your physician before beginning a new exercise program.

To perform the workouts in this book, I recommend the following equipment:

- A stability (exercise) ball (55 to 75 centimeters)

- 3 pairs of dumbbells: light, medium, and heavy

- A foam roller (you can use a tennis ball or rolling pin if you are on a budget)

- An exercise step (or sturdy step stool)

Do you belong to a gym? If so, it should have these tools. If you plan to buy equipment and work out on your own, use this guideline for dumbbells. Start with a moderate weight dumbbell, 8-12 pounds for women and 12-20 pounds for men. Perform dumbbell biceps curls and count how many you can do.

If you can do more than 16-20 repetitions (reps), this will be your light pair of dumbbells. If you can do between 12-16 reps, this is your medium pair: Buy one pair the next heavier weight and one pair the next lighter weight from your original medium pair of dumbbells. If you can do at most between 6-12 repetitions, this is your heavy pair; buy two additional pairs (two weight selections lighter than your heavy pair). These exercise tools are excellent to start you on your fitness journey.

You can also practice more of the Phase II workouts with these optional tools:

- BOSU ball (blue half-dome balance ball)

- One 8-16 pound medicine ball

- Ankle and/or wrist weights

- Cardio machine like a treadmill or an elliptical

- Exercise mat (you can use a thick towel if you do not want to buy a mat)

Heart rate zones are different levels of intensity for your heart. These zones determine what source of fuel your body uses during exercise. Your body mostly uses either fat or glucose (carbohydrates) as fuel sources.

There are also methods of monitoring your heart rate by using a perceived rate of exertion. Refer to the appendix for a chart on "perceived rate of exertion."

### What Is Cardio?

Cardiovascular (cardio) exercise is defined by raising your heart rate to zone 1 (or higher) or 65% of your maximum heart rate. See Heart Rate Zones later in this chapter to figure out if you are doing physical activity or cardiovascular exercise. If you are not sure how to check your heart rate, use the Perceived Rate of Exertion chart in the appendix.

- Heart rate monitor—this is helpful to get an accurate account of your heart rate zones and to find out how many calories you burn during exercise

Again, if you belong to a fitness center, most of these tools should be available for use or for sale. If not, feel free to request them. You may not be the only person looking for a foam roller, but you may be the only person to ask!

## Physical Activity versus Cardiovascular Training (Cardio Training)

You should move your body every day. This is no news flash, but even though the benefits are so immense, we still choose to do more sitting than moving. Create habits to get you active every day. Examples of physical activity include:

- Walking—take a family (or pet) walk before dinner every night

- Dancing—do this after dinner while cleaning the kitchen. Turn on your favorite music and dance while you work!

- Playing recreational sports—look for adult recreation teams in your community: volleyball, softball, golf, et cetera. These adult sports are a great way to get active and meet people in your community with similar interests!

- Raking leaves—make leaf houses with the neighbor kids

- Light house cleaning—need I say more? Do not forget the music!

This type of movement keeps our joints lubricated, increases circulation, and prevents arthritis; these benefits are an active recipe for physical longevity. *Cardiovascular training is different*; it is more intense than light physical activity.

Cardio training or exercise is defined as exercise that gets your heart rate up to at least 65% of your maximum heart rate (imagine a run versus a walk around the block). This type of training strengthens your heart and prevents diseases like heart disease, high blood pressure, and diabetes. Cardio exercise is also a great way to achieve and maintain a healthy weight. Cardio training zones can be measured by first figuring out your heart rate zones.

## Calculating Your Heart Rate Zones

How do you calculate your heart rate zones? Below is a simple way to find your maximum heart rate and your approximate heart rate zones. Heart rate zones are math equations; they show how to monitor how hard your heart is working. If you were training for a specific event, I would recommend using the Karvonen Method (not shown), which factors in your resting heart rate.

Calculating your heart rate (cardio) zones:
What is your age? _____

Max Heart Rate (MHR): 220 -_____= _____ (age) (MHR)

Zone 1= 65-75% of your MHR: _____ (You should feel in control–you could stay in this zone for more than two hours.)

Zone 2 = 76-85% of your MHR: _____ (You should feel challenged–you could hold for the majority of your cardio workout here for twenty minutes to two hours.)

Zone 3 = 86-95% MHR: _____ (You should feel as though you want out–you could *not* hold this for more than two minutes.)

Remember, it is important to have an understanding of your heart rate zones so that you know if you are working hard enough to meet your goals or if you are working too hard and overtraining your heart. To improve your current fitness level, the National Academy of Sports Medicine recommends adding a minimum of thirty minutes per day, three to five times per week of cardiovascular exercise. Several short cardio workouts (ten- to fifteen minute spurts at different times in one day) can be just as effective as one long cardio workout. Again, this is different from light physical activity. Below are some examples of cardio training activities:

• Cycling • Jumping Rope • Running (4-6 mph) • Rowing (fast) • Mountain Biking • Swimming • Elliptical Training • Skiing • Weight Lifting

## Two Birds. One Dumbbell? Cardio and Strength Together

Cardio and strength training can be accomplished simultaneously. Circuit training is performing one strength exercise after another with minimal rest in between exercises. This type of training keeps your *heart rate elevated for the duration of the workout*. The workouts in this book may be performed as a circuit if they are executed with minimal rest in between exercises.

**Figuring out Percentages**

Below is an example of how to find a percent of your maximum heart rate (MHR).

To figure out 65% of a number, take the number and multiply it by 0.65.

**Two birds. One dumbbell. Why I love circuit training:**

Circuit training breaks up mundane routines: Moving quickly from one exercise to the next keeps your body and your mind engaged.

An all-strength circuit burns 30% more calories (about 9 calories per minute!) than a typical strength training workout and offers more cardio benefits because your heart rate is elevated the entire workout.

A workout that combines cardio and strength will blast fat and sculpt your muscles.

How many times this week do you plan to practice cardio exercise?

Who can you ask (a buddy) to exercise with you?

What is your exercise backup plan (Examples: workout with a DVD indoors if it rains or turn on some music and dance)?

**What Is Interval Training?**

Interval training is an effective form of cardio and/or strength that challenges your heart rate in all three zones several times in one workout. Interval training is an effective way to build cardiovascular strength and endurance.

High intensity interval training is introduced in Phase Three of this book (Power Level). High-intensity interval training helps you break through plateaus. However, your body needs a strong foundation and core stabilization before you train your muscles this way. Be sure to follow the workouts in progression for injury prevention.

# Share to Learn (S2L)

By sharing information, ideas, thoughts, and feelings with someone or a group of people, *you* have a unique opportunity to learn and become more grounded from teaching the information you just learned.

If you are reading this book with a group of friends as a small group study (which I highly recommend), reading it by yourself, or reading it with one close friend, I strongly encourage you to participate in the S2L sections. Give sharing a try. Sharing information from a field where you are not the expert (yet) might feel strange. But this exercise of teaching someone one or two pieces of information you just read is a vital part of retaining what you learned, seeking accountability, and learning from someone else in community (together). Furthermore, we need each other to unearth what is on our hearts. We cannot journey this life on our own and have any lasting meaning. *One purpose in pursuing optimal health is not to be interrupted by preventable diseases.* Give sharing a try—you have everything to gain!

# S2L

Share with someone (or discuss in your small group) what the definition of health is according to Don Colbert, MD, and the World Health Organization and then make up your own definition of health and explain your ideas.

What is your definition of health?

_____

_____


Discuss the importance of understanding the function of calories.

Approximately how many calories do you need per day to achieve your weight goals? _____

Describe your fitness goals and your plan of how to achieve them. Tell someone how many times you are going to exercise per week, what time of day, and what your backup plan is if your first option falls through:

_____

_____


With whom are you going to discuss your thoughts, goals, and ideas?

_____

_____

# Time to Get InFIT!

## Stabilization. Strength. Power.
## InFIT Workout Guidelines

The workouts in this book follow the National Academy of Sports Medicine Optimum Performance Training™ (OPT) training model guidelines. This proven method begins with exercises that promote stabilization, move to exercises that promote strength, and finish with exercises that promote power training. Because of the progression of exercises, each workout should be practiced one to three times per week over a one- to four-week period. Be sure to give your muscles forty-eight hours of rest between strength workouts for adequate repair before working the same muscle group again. Example: If you perform InFIT Workout 1 on Monday, wait until Wednesday or Thursday to do Workout 1 again. Repeat the same workout at least three times before moving on to the next chapter's workout (repetition builds a strong foundation).

In the Stabilization Endurance Level, the full-body, strength-training workouts are meant to be performed circuit style with one exercise from each row (lower body, upper body, and core) with minimal rest between exercises. Repeat the pattern with the next column. You can go through the warmup, all nine exercises, and stretching one time (one set) in approximately twenty to twenty-five minutes. If you want to increase your strength gains faster, or you want to focus on a specific muscle group, keep repeating the exercises of your choice to complete additional sets. The more you work your muscles, the faster you will see definition and weight loss results. If you have not worked out in at least a month, set small, attainable goals. Developing lasting habits are much easier when your goals are realistic and your practice is consistent. You can always increase your exercise with time, but it is more difficult to get back on the path if you become burnt out or injured.

> ### Listen to Your Body!
>
> As the workouts progress in difficulty, make sure you are listening to your body. If a particular exercise or workout causes pain to your joints, skip it and move to the next (or previous) exercise or workout.
>
> If the next phase is too difficult, stay in your current phase until you feel more comfortable advancing.
>
> InFIT Workouts are designed for you to get stronger, more flexible, and more balanced. Never compromise proper form on an exercise that is too difficult.
>
> The quality of your workouts is far more important than the quantity. A focused 20 minutes is better than a sloppy 2 hours.

## Stabilization Endurance Level

During the Stabilization Endurance Level (InFIT Workouts 1-4), we work on:

- Improving your muscular endurance

- Enhancing your joint stability

- Increasing your flexibility

- Enhancing control of your posture

- Improving your neuromuscular efficiency (balance and stabilization together)

The goal in the Stabilization Endurance Level is to fatigue (exhaust the muscle) after no more than 20 repetitions (reps). If you can do more than 20 reps per exercise, increase your weight or move to Option II exercises with the same guidelines, as the exercises in Option II are more challenging.

## Strength Level

During the Strength Level (InFIT Workouts 5-8), we continue building on the foundation you developed in the Stabilization Endurance Level. The benefits in the Strength Level include the following:

- Improving your stabilization endurance, increasing prime mover (main muscle) strength and volume of training

- Increasing the ability of your core to stabilize your spine and pelvis

- Enhancing stability in your joints, ligaments, muscles, and tendons

- Increasing your lean body mass, bone mineral density, and weight loss

The goal in the Strength Level is to fatigue your muscles after no more than 12 reps. In this level, we will transition from performing one exercise in each row, to performing all three exercises in the same row before moving on to the next muscle group (lower body, upper body, and core). This progression of exercises is called supersetting. If you can do more than 12 reps per exercise, increase your weight or move to Option II exercises with the same guidelines.

## Power Level

During the Power Level (InFIT Workouts 9-12), we focus on both high force and velocity to develop muscles that can dynamically move in all planes of motion. Combining strength exercises with power exercises on the same muscle group, we continue the supersetting pattern. If the exercise says "speed" in the description, you will use light resistance with a fast tempo, 8-10 reps each. If the exercise does not indicate "speed" in the description, you will use heavy resistance with an explosive tempo, 5-10 reps each.

The benefits of power training include the following:

- Enhancing your neuromuscular efficiency

- Enhancing your prime mover strength and speed strength

- Increasing your rate of force production (power)

- Enhancing your lean body mass, bone mineral density, and weight loss

The goal in the Power Level is to fatigue after no more than 10 reps. If you can do more than 10 reps per exercise, increase your weight or move to Option II exercises with the same guidelines. After completing all the exercises in the Power Level, cycle back through Levels 1 and 2 for a minimum of four weeks each.

## Self-Myofascial Release (SMR) and Stretching

Self-myofascial release is another word for foam rolling, a flexibility technique that applies pressure from a piece of cylinder-shaped foam to an adhesion or knot in your muscle. To perform foam rolling, apply gentle pressure to the knot for a minimum of thirty seconds (see pictures for details in the stretching instruction section in this chapter). Once the knot is released, your muscles may return to their optimum length, preventing injuries and allowing for a full range of motion. *Please allow time for foam rolling and stretching!* Static stretching your muscles (taking the muscle to tension and holding with low force) is also as important as the workout itself for injury prevention, proper posture, and muscle, joint, and bone health. In addition to foam rolling, static stretching should be held for at least thirty seconds to allow your muscles to relax and hold their length.

According to the National Academy of Sports Medicine, research suggests you should stretch tight muscles before and after you work out. Stretching tight muscles before you work out may enhance your activity by allowing for a full range of motion. Please refer back to the stretching instruction page in this chapter for a full range of foam roll and stretching exercises. Consult with a personal trainer to assess which muscles are inhibited, or select stretching exercises that coincide with the muscles you have just worked or tight muscles.

## Progress Is Motivating!

Track your progress. Record the weight you used (if applicable), how many repetitions (reps) you performed, and how many times you repeated the exercise (sets) in the boxes below the exercise descriptions. Remember your goals; seeing your progress will help you stay motivated and focused on your fitness journey! Use the examples below to help you fill out your own exercise boxes:

*Front Lunge to Balance*   *Front Lunge to Balance*

| Weight | 12lbs |  |
|--------|-------|--|
| Sets | 2 | |
| Reps | 20 | |

| Weight | 12lbs | 15lbs |
|--------|-------|-------|
| Sets | 2 | 2 |
| Reps | 20 | 24 |

Use the second column in the exercise box to record your weight, sets, and reps the first time you practice the exercise. Next time you work out (and perform the same exercise), use the third column to record changes in your variables.

## Hydration

Finally, stay hydrated! Your muscles need water to perform and your cells need water to deliver nutrients to your heart and lungs. In addition to the regular amount of water you need per day (half of your ideal body weight in ounces), you should consume an extra 20 ounces for every hour of exercise you perform. For a whole page of tasty vitamin water recipes, see Chapter 10. Get your water bottle and get off the couch!

### Water

Drinking half of your ideal body weight in ounces is recommended per day.

What is considered water?

Water is any liquid without added sugar, artificial sweeteners, caffeine, or calories.

Coffee does not count toward your water intake because it contains caffeine, which is a diuretic (dehydrates your body). Decaf does not count either. Water contains no added chemicals.

## Practice

1. Keep a wellness journal. Make it personal by writing important objectives for your health, nutrition, exercise, sleep, body composition, feelings, successes, challenges, et cetera. If you track your nutrition electronically, I encourage you to keep a separate wellness journal on a computer or notebook. Take this opportunity to get to know your body and yourself better.

2. Make a plan. How often are you going to work out?

What time of day are you going to work out?

3. What is your backup plan?

## 12-Week InFIT Workout Plan

Copy or print this sample workout plan and put it near your calendar. To stay accountable and build momentum in your fitness routine, cross off workouts once they have been completed. Feel free to modify this plan as much as you desire. If it looks too intimidating, make it your goal to complete half the workouts until you have developed a consistent routine. When you are ready, add additional days to your plan. Remember, one or two short bursts of exercise can be as effective as one long workout per day. You can start with three minutes or thirty minutes. *The important part is that you start!* After you complete your 12-Week InFIT Workout Plan, repeat the program, beginning with InFIT Workout 1–Option II (use InFIT Workouts Option II on your strength days for the next twelve weeks). Continue alternating between Option I and Option II workouts every twelve weeks. Increase your weight, reps, and sets as needed for optimal strength gains (toning) and/or body fat reduction (weight loss).

### Stabilization Endurance Level

| | Workout | Monday | Tuesday | Wednesday | Thursday | Friday | Saturday | Sunday |
|---|---|---|---|---|---|---|---|---|
| **Week 1** | InFIT Workout 1 on Strength Days | Cardio | Strength | Cardio | Strength | Cardio | Strength | Light activity or rest day |
| **Week 2** | InFIT Workout 2 on Strength Days | Strength | Cardio | Strength | Cardio | Strength | Cardio | Light activity or rest day |
| **Week 3** | InFIT Workout 3 on Strength Days | Cardio | Strength | Cardio | Strength | Cardio | Strength | Light activity or rest day |
| **Week 4** | InFIT Workout 4 on Strength Days | Strength | Cardio | Strength | Cardio | Strength | Cardio | Light activity or rest day |

## Strength Level

| | Workout | Monday | Tuesday | Wednesday | Thursday | Friday | Saturday | Sunday |
|---|---|---|---|---|---|---|---|---|
| Week 1 | InFIT Workout 5 on Strength Days | Cardio | Strength | Cardio | Strength | Cardio | Strength | Light activity or rest day |
| Week 2 | InFIT Workout 6 on Strength Days | Strength | Cardio | Strength | Cardio | Strength | Cardio | Light activity or rest day |
| Week 3 | InFIT Workout 7 on Strength Days | Cardio | Strength | Cardio | Strength | Cardio | Strength | Light activity or rest day |
| Week 4 | InFIT Workout 8 on Strength Days | Strength | Cardio | Strength | Cardio | Strength | Cardio | Light activity or rest day |

## Power Level

| | Workout | Monday | Tuesday | Wednesday | Thursday | Friday | Saturday | Sunday |
|---|---|---|---|---|---|---|---|---|
| Week 1 | InFIT Workout 9 on Strength Days | Cardio | Strength | Cardio | Strength | Cardio | Strength | Light activity or rest day |
| Week 2 | InFIT Workout 10 on Strength Days | Strength | Cardio | Strength | Cardio | Strength | Cardio | Light activity or rest day |
| Week 3 | InFIT Workout 11 on Strength Days | Cardio | Strength | Cardio | Strength | Cardio | Strength | Light activity or rest day |
| Week 4 | InFIT Workout 12 on Strength Days | Strength | Cardio | Strength | Cardio | Strength | Cardio | Light activity or rest day |

## Notes

_____

_____

_____

_____

_____

_____

_____

_____

_____

# InFIT Workout 1

**First time (set) through:** Warm up. Go through all of the exercises slowly, 15-20 repetitions (reps) each, with no resistance (no weight), 3-5 minutes. **Second set:** Perform the exercises one at a time, with resistance when appropriate, starting with one lower body exercise, one upper body exercise, and one core exercise with minimal rest in between. Perform all nine exercises and then repeat as your fitness goals and time permit! Phase I is designed to build your body's stabilization endurance, core strength, and to prepare you for more challenging moves in the future. Take your time working through the exercises. Usually, slower is better (and safer, too). Remember to stretch your muscles as stretching is as important as the workout itself.

## Lower Body

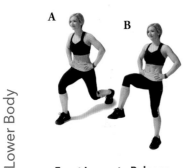

**Front Lunge to Balance**

|  | Set 1 | Set 2 |
|---|---|---|
| **Weight** |  |  |
| **Reps** |  |  |

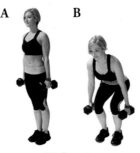

**DB Squat**

|  | Set 1 | Set 2 |
|---|---|---|
| **Weight** |  |  |
| **Reps** |  |  |

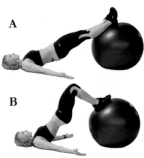

**SB Hamstring Curl**

|  | Set 1 | Set 2 |
|---|---|---|
| **Weight** |  |  |
| **Reps** |  |  |

## Upper Body

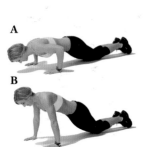

**Knee Pushup**

|  | Set 1 | Set 2 |
|---|---|---|
| **Weight** |  |  |
| **Reps** |  |  |

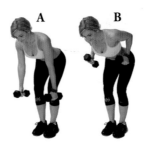

**DB Bent Over Row**

|  | Set 1 | Set 2 |
|---|---|---|
| **Weight** |  |  |
| **Reps** |  |  |

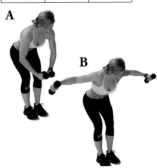

**DB Bent Over Reverse Fly**

|  | Set 1 | Set 2 |
|---|---|---|
| **Weight** |  |  |
| **Reps** |  |  |

## Core

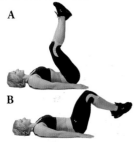

**Leg Lift with Bent Knees**

|  | Set 1 | Set 2 |
|---|---|---|
| **Weight** |  |  |
| **Reps** |  |  |

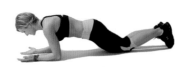

**Prone Plank**

|  | Set 1 | Set 2 |
|---|---|---|
| **Weight** |  |  |
| **Reps** |  |  |

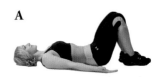
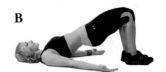

**Bridge–Double Leg**

|  | Set 1 | Set 2 |
|---|---|---|
| **Weight** |  |  |
| **Reps** |  |  |

# InFIT Workout 1–Option II

Option II is designed for you if you have been working out consistently (with a certified personal trainer if possible) for at least one month. Perform the exercises one at a time starting with one lower body exercise, one upper body exercise, then one core exercise with minimal rest in between. Perform all nine exercises and then repeat as your fitness goals and time permit! Remember to stretch your muscles as stretching is as important as the workout itself.

**Lower Body**

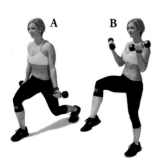

### DB Front Lunge to Balance with Biceps Curl

|  | Set 1 | Set 2 |
|---|---|---|
| **Weight** |  |  |
| **Reps** |  |  |

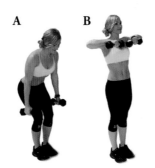

### DB Squat to Upright Row

|  | Set 1 | Set 2 |
|---|---|---|
| **Weight** |  |  |
| **Reps** |  |  |

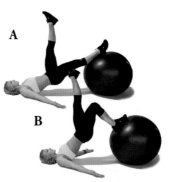

### SB Single Leg Hamstring Curl

|  | Set 1 | Set 2 |
|---|---|---|
| **Weight** |  |  |
| **Reps** |  |  |

**Upper Body**

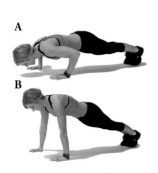

### Full Body Pushup

|  | Set 1 | Set 2 |
|---|---|---|
| **Weight** |  |  |
| **Reps** |  |  |

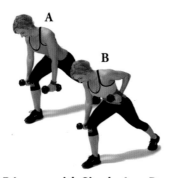

### DB Lunge with Single Arm Row

|  | Set 1 | Set 2 |
|---|---|---|
| **Weight** |  |  |
| **Reps** |  |  |

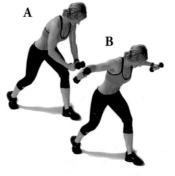

### DB Lunge with Reverse Fly

|  | Set 1 | Set 2 |
|---|---|---|
| **Weight** |  |  |
| **Reps** |  |  |

**Core**

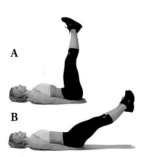

### Leg Lift with Straight Legs

|  | Set 1 | Set 2 |
|---|---|---|
| **Weight** |  |  |
| **Reps** |  |  |

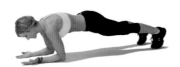

### Prone Plank on Toes

|  | Set 1 | Set 2 |
|---|---|---|
| **Weight** |  |  |
| **Reps** |  |  |

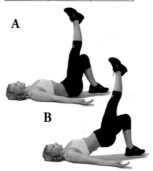

### Bridge–Single Leg

|  | Set 1 | Set 2 |
|---|---|---|
| **Weight** |  |  |
| **Reps** |  |  |

# Foam Rolling and Stretching

Please allow time for foam rolling (self-myofascial release) and stretching! Flexibility is vital for injury prevention and muscle, joint, and bone health. According to the National Academy of Sports Medicine, research suggests that you can stretch before and after your workout. Stretching before you work out is *not* stretching cold muscles, as previously thought by fitness professionals. Light, static (holding, never bouncing) stretches and foam rolling before you begin may enhance your workout by eliminating tight muscles and allowing for a full range of motion during your workout. *Please refer back to this page after each workout for a full range of foam roll and stretching exercises.* If you do not have time to perform all the stretches, select stretching exercises that coincide with the muscles you just exercised and muscles that are tight. Hold each stretch for at least 30 seconds or 5-7 full breaths.

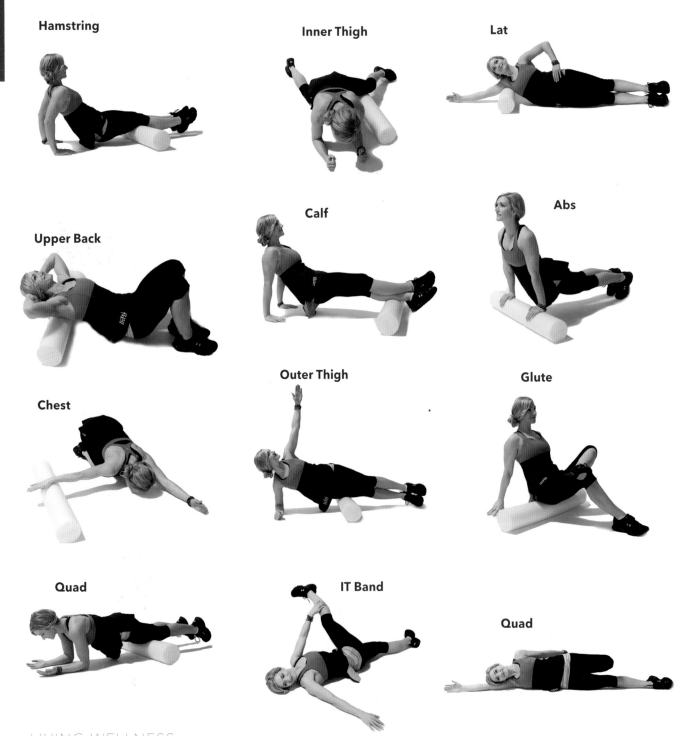

**Hamstring**

**Inner Thigh**

**Lat**

**Upper Back**

**Calf**

**Abs**

**Chest**

**Outer Thigh**

**Glute**

**Quad**

**IT Band**

**Quad**

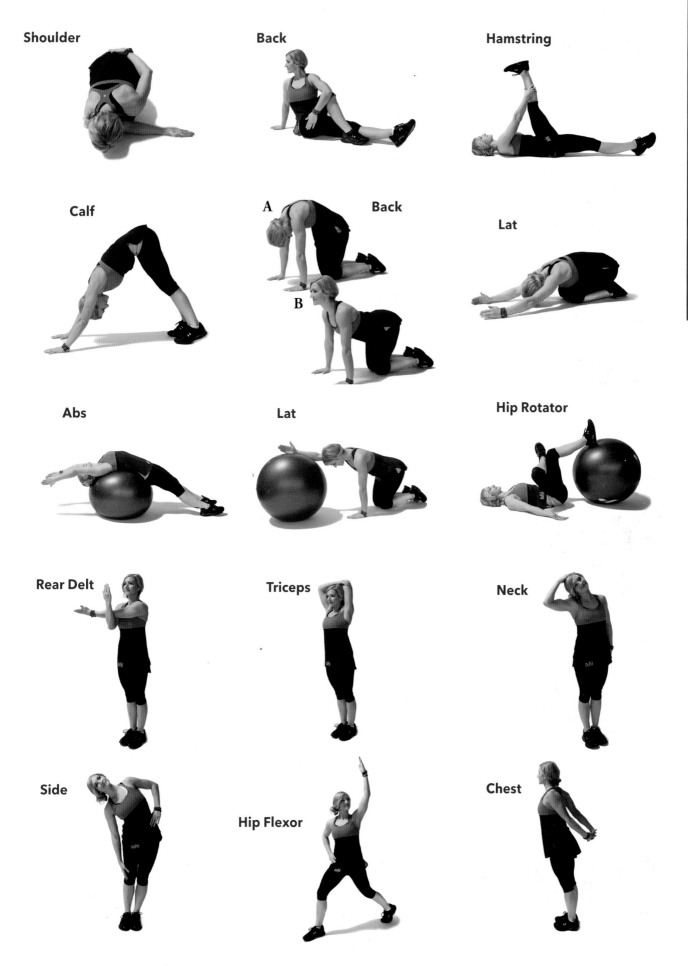

Shoulder

Back

Hamstring

Calf

**A** Back

**B**

Lat

Abs

Lat

Hip Rotator

Rear Delt

Triceps

Neck

Side

Hip Flexor

Chest

## Review Your Map—Chapter Reflection

Use this road map as a weekly check-in to measure your goals and progress. Fill in the blank spaces at the bottom of the chart to create your own goals. The more often you check in with yourself, the more often you will bring health to the front of your mind, creating intention and success.

| | GOAL | MON Actual | TUE Actual | WED Actual | THU Actual | FRI Actual | SAT Actual | SUN Actual |
|---|---|---|---|---|---|---|---|---|
| Servings of produce (Ch 5) | | | | | | | | |
| Water in ounces | | | | | | | | |
| Hours of sleep (Ch 2) | | | | | | | | |
| Minutes of exercise | | | | | | | | |
| Weight | | | | | | | | |
| Amount of meals/ snacks per day (Ch 3) | | | | | | | | |
| Calories | | | | | | | | |
| Number of simple carbs (Ch 6) | | | | | | | | |
| Body fat % (optional) | | | | | | | | |
| Bowel movements (Ch 8) | | | | | | | | |
| Add your own below | | | | | | | | |
| | | | | | | | | |
| | | | | | | | | |
| | | | | | | | | |

Did you achieve most of your goals? _____ Why? _____

What is your plan for the next week to either stay on your original course or modify based on this week's review?

How do you feel about your progress thus far?

# LIVING AFFIRMATION
## WELLNESS FOR YOUR SOUL

## Welcome! Introduction to the Living Affirmations

A warm and excited welcome from me, Christina, to this fantastic guidebook that can change every aspect of your life!

I look at the physical body as the temple of the Holy Spirit, who empowers us from within. The body is not only relevant in the physical realm but also as an expression of what is going on in the unseen, spiritual realm. Without the soul, the body dies, and without the body, the soul's purpose on earth is useless. Therefore we must take good care of both the body and the soul because they are fully connected. *My passion and sense of responsibility for optimal nutrition and fitness come from understanding the connectedness between our bodies and souls.*

Many people think of the physical body as a mere "temporary container," inferior to the soul. Out of that mindset flows the attitude that we do not need to pay much attention to the body, that we can stuff it with whatever food comes into our hands, and ignore the body's need for daily physical activity. For example, since immigrating from Germany to the United States in 2010, I have been to numerous community and church potlucks that are as nutrient-void and calorie-laden as common fast food. We cannot lead our lives in ignorance about the connected role of physical and spiritual health.

The society of the Western world, including the church, is struck by obesity, disease, and sickness. We are weakened and distracted by sicknesses resulting directly from our lifestyle choices.

In each affirmation I will offer you "food for the soul." My hope is that these affirmations will inspire you to think more profoundly about the health of your body and your soul. I encourage you to share what you discover with a friend.

Be blessed abundantly! ~ *Christina Zaczkowski*, MA, CPT

## *Reflection*

_____

_____

_____

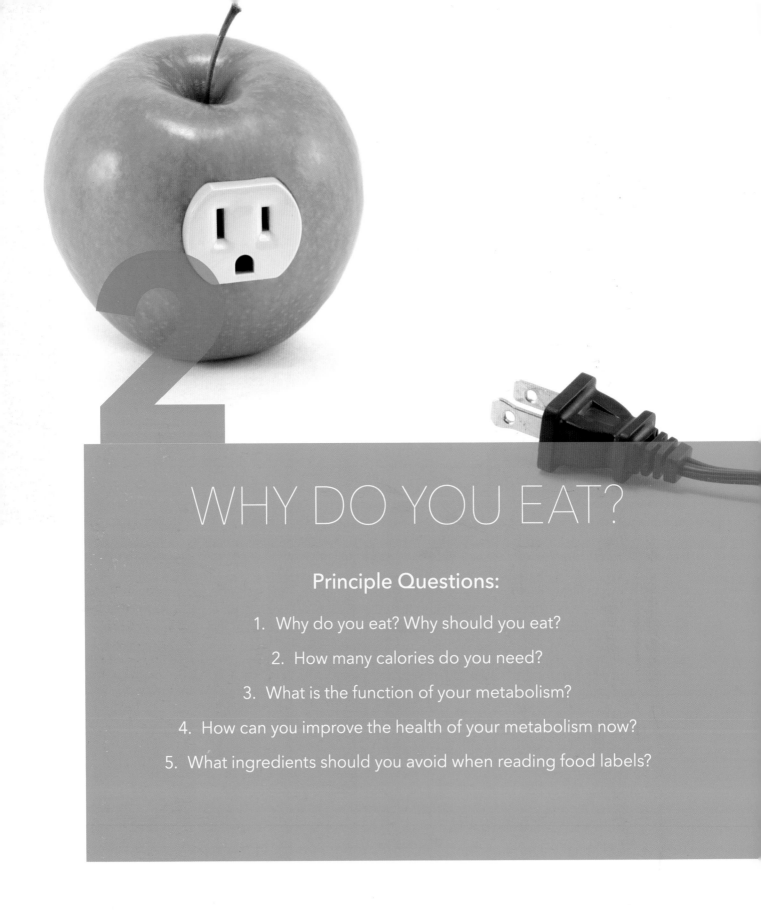

# WHY DO YOU EAT?

### Principle Questions:

1. Why do you eat? Why should you eat?

2. How many calories do you need?

3. What is the function of your metabolism?

4. How can you improve the health of your metabolism now?

5. What ingredients should you avoid when reading food labels?

**W**hy do you eat? Why should you eat? Are these two questions the same? No, definitely not.

The biggest challenge with wellness and weight management is not a problem with a *lack* of information. We are in the information age. Google search *What should I eat?* and you will be bombarded with services and products to buy, including meal ideas, recipes, diets, diet pills, and programs for menu planning. The Center for Disease Control (CDC) has an entire program devoted to what we should eat (MyPlate), which we will look at in Chapter 5. My experience has shown that *moving more and eating less results in weight loss*. But if it were that easy, why do so many of us struggle with weight?

*Here are two main challenges (amongst many more):*

- You are busy.

- You are distracted.

Am I right? You might be familiar with thoughts like: I know I need to *eat more produce and less fast food,* but where do I find the time to prepare healthy food? I know I need to *drink less soda and drink more water,* but how will I get though the day with no energy? I know that I should *eat clean foods and less processed foods,* but what should I look for on food labels?

The topics in this book are earth shattering. They are proven, effective, and realistic. *My plea for you:* Do not give up on yourself.

My favorite idea about health and wellness is that you are never too far off the wagon to turn around and jump back on! Read this book every day. Do the worksheets. Do the practice sections. Even if you put this book down for a season or two, pick it back up and start again. The goal of *Living Wellness* is not to stuff knowledge in your mind. Instead, the goal of *Living Wellness* is to keep your priorities top of mind so that the habits you create stay with you until they become natural, like tying your shoes and brushing your teeth.

Because persistence is so important, let me repeat my plea: *Do not give up on yourself.*

Keep this book close, on your nightstand or at your work desk.

Health and wellness has to be *top of mind*, an intentional decision. Do not expect good health to happen on its own. However, know that it *will* improve with your intentional decisions.

Now, for the meat (or veggies if you prefer), why do you eat?

Individuals eat for a variety of reasons: hunger, thirst, anxiety, joy, boredom, self-soothing, guilt, social engagements, memories, et cetera. I used to eat mindlessly when I was excited or anxious about something.

Why do you eat?

Why should you eat?

Do you have food triggers (any reasons for eating other than for fuel or nourishment)?

How can you comfort yourself with something other than food?

The goal of *Living Wellness* is not to stuff knowledge in your mind.

The goal of *Living Wellness* is to keep your priorities top of mind so that the habits you create stay with you until they become natural, like tying your shoes and brushing your teeth.

# Why *Should* You eat?

1. Fuel

2. Nourishment

3. Pleasure (We have taste buds, right?)

But, Ashley, are fuel and nourishment the same? Well, no. You can get *fuel* from a candy bar, but you are sure not getting a lot of nourishment. Conversely, you can get *nourishment* from a calcium supplement, but you are not going to get any fuel. Do you see the difference? Why, then, should you eat? You should eat for fuel *and* nourishment (and pleasure).

**Do you overeat?**

Yes/No

Why ?

*"The saddest thing, I think, amongst all common but tragic ironies, is to feel fat and very hungry at the same time."*

Unknown

## Food as Fuel

For fuel, we need a certain amount of calories (energy) per day to maintain our bodily systems such as respiratory, circulatory, cardiovascular, lymphatic, digestive, skeletal, endocrine, muscular, immune, and nervous systems. Calories provide fuel for our bodies.

Too many calories result in weight gain and too few calories (or the wrong kind of calories) result in malnourishment. Exceptions include certain metabolic disorders that need to be treated medically. Check with your doctor if you think you have a metabolic disorder. However, most people with metabolic disorders can still manage their wellness and weight under the care of health and fitness professionals.

## Overeating

If you fill your car's tank with fuel and keep pumping even after it is filled, where does the extra go? In addition to wasting money and resources, the extra fuel will flow out of the tank and make a mess on the ground. Fortunately and unfortunately, our bodies have a similar overflow outage. When we overeat, the excess fuel turns into fat and fills the cells already in our bodies, making them larger. As we continue to overeat, the fat cells grow larger, *or* if we gain a significant amount of weight, the body produces *more cells* to store the excess body fat. A dangerous sign of overconsuming carbohydrates or added sugar is excessive glucose from carbohydrates overflowing into the urine, which is a symptom of diabetes.

Understanding the process of overeating brings to light the importance of having enough (without excess) fuel for our bodies to function properly. Having adequate energy to get through the day feeling good and desiring to be active with our family and friends allows us to enjoy and engage in life, rather than feel sluggish from a lack of fuel (starvation mode from not eating enough calories) or lethargic from the wrong type of fuel (junk food, processed food, food high in sugar or sodium).

# How Many Calories Do You Need?

Everyone is different. Refer to Chapter 1 for a formula to figure out your basal metabolic rate (BMR) and an estimate of maintenance calories based on your age and weight. Then record it here for quick reference:

BMR: _____   Maintenance calories: _____

Goal calories: _____

A baseline recommendation of 2,000 calories is not suitable for everyone. Think about all the different shapes, sizes, and activity levels of all the people in the world; there is a lot of variance.

If you commute a long distance to work or school every day, your vehicle is going to need more fuel than if you were to commute only a few miles every day. Your body works the same way. The less active you are, the less fuel you need.

## Size Matters

If you have a sedentary job or you are limited in your daily physical activity, you may need far fewer calories than someone who works in physical construction or someone who waits tables. If you are a petite person like myself, you probably need far fewer calories than your counterpart. This might mean that you have to exercise more discipline at meals and in social settings. Also, there are vehicles and fuel types that are much more efficient in their mileage than other vehicles. The same is true of our fuel:

- Better fuel from food choices equals more efficiency (faster metabolism).

- Better fuel from food choices equals cleaner burning (better health).

Remember, a 3,500-calorie surplus or deficit equals 1 pound of body fat gained or lost, respectively.

Let us review an example of how to formulate a goal calorie range to avoid overfilling our bodies with fuel:

Based on the calorie calculator in Chapter 1, our forty-five-year-old female needs 1,672 calories to maintain her current weight. She would like to lose 1-2 pounds of body fat per week.

- 1,672 calories a day to maintain her current weight

- MINUS 500 calorie deficit per day (reduced food calories)

- 1,172 calories per day consumed for 1 pound of body fat loss per week

- MINUS 500 calories per day in exercise

### What Is "Starvation Mode"?

As the name suggests, your body goes into starvation mode when you skip meals—breakfast included! Your body needs refueling every three to four hours. Especially after sleeping for six or more hours, you need to *break* the *fast* and enjoy a healthy breakfast rather than sprinting out the door or saving the calories for later. Besides the psychological effects of skipping meals, your body hangs on to the calories from your next meal as a protective mechanism to avoid "starvation."

*Let us see the scale for what it is: a measure of how much you weigh, not a measure of your worth.*

- *672 NET calories per day to lose 2 pounds of body fat per week*

- A 1,000-calorie deficit per day through food and beverage (calorie reduction) and exercise will result in 2 pounds per week of body fat loss.

## Undereating

I have had clients ask me if they can just consume 672 calories per day to lose 2 pounds per week in order to avoid exercise. The answer is no. *This severe calorie deficit is not healthy* and consequently, there is no way to get enough nourishment. See a nutritionist or doctor if you want an exact number (which varies slightly every day). It is generally accepted that women should not consume fewer than approximately 1,200 calories per day and men should not consume fewer than approximately 1,800 per day. Remember you need fuel *and* nourishment, and if you consume too few calories, you are not nourishing your body.

You must take good care of your metabolism for the above calorie formula to work. You are already learning how to take good care by reading this book. Let us look at how to fuel your metabolism so it works on your behalf (by burning fat) rather than against you (by storing fat).

## What Is the Function of Your Metabolism?

The chemistry behind your metabolism is complicated. Think of your metabolism as the stoplights and law enforcement in a city, carefully regulating the flow of traffic to maintain peace much like your body chemistry (metabolism) constantly regulating chemicals and hormones to maintain balance. According to an article from the Mayo Clinic, your metabolism is responsible for breaking down, digesting, absorbing, transporting, and storing or burning the food you consume. There are many moving parts in an efficient traffic flow and in a healthy metabolism.

*No one has perfect eating habits. Let's not make that our goal. Let's make our goal be to eat cleaner and healthier than we did yesterday.*

### When Should You Stop Eating?

You should finish eating at least two hours before bedtime. This increases sleep quality, cellular repair, and sets the stage for optimal fat burning while you sleep, so you wake up feeling lighter and ready to *break* the *fast*!

It is easy to blame weight gain on a slow metabolism, but the concept of a slow metabolism does not exist. Your metabolism is a chemistry lab, not a drag race. Unless you have a metabolic disorder, *weight gain is a result of consuming more calories than your body needs—usually because the calories we consume are void of nutritional value, causing you to eat more.*

We may feel like our metabolism keeps us looking to sugar for energy to get up and go, *but usually the sugar we eat damages the stoplights of our metabolism.* Consuming added sugar turns on the *red light* for burning fat as fuel. But complex carbohydrates, like vegetables, turn on the *green light* for burning fat as fuel. The foods we eat, how often we eat, how much water we drink, how much muscle we have, how much sleep we get, and how often we exercise affect the flow of our metabolism.

You can improve the chemistry of your metabolism *today*. You can make small, effective changes that *will* impact how you look and feel instantly. Eventually, your body composition will reflect your new choices.

# Boost Your Metabolism Right Now

**Eat breakfast and small frequent meals every three to four hours.** You would not expect your vehicle to run without fuel and you should not expect your body to either. Breakfast is meant to *break* the *fast*. I hope that you went to bed with an empty stomach and your body is ready to eat and be energized in the morning. You should eat something healthy within one hour of waking. If breakfast upsets your stomach, try something with less acid (an egg rather than orange juice, for example). After breakfast, you should *eat small frequent meals or snacks every three to four hours*; a couple of hundred calories each depending on your caloric needs. We will examine specifics in Chapter 3 regarding what you should eat.

**Water, Water, Water.** One study published in the *Journal of Clinical Endocrinology and Metabolism* reports that drinking 17 ounces of water (preferably filtered) in one sitting increases metabolic rate by 30%! Your body uses *calories* to process water. Remember, you should be drinking approximately half of your ideal body weight in ounces every day. Water is responsible for bringing nutrients into and removing waste from every cell. Water also aids in digestion, balances body fluids, helps you feel full, keeps your muscles energized, keeps your skin elastic, and flushes your kidneys and liver. Imagine putting yesterday's lunch in a blender. How would your blender sound when you turned it on? Now, imagine adding 20 ounces of water to the blender—the contents would digest better. Our stomach and our digestive tract need water, as does every cell in our bodies.

**Your plate.** Again, imagine all of yesterday's food in a blender. Would it blend smoothly if it was full of simple carbohydrates like muffins, hamburger buns, crackers, candy, and pizza crust? Intestines and bowels filled with too many simple carbohydrates get clogged, jammed, and constipated. Half of your plate at every meal should be fruits and veggies. Slightly more than a quarter of your plate should be protein, and the rest should be complex carbohydrates and whole grains. Your plate should also be dressed with healthy fat, which we will discuss in Chapter 7. (We will talk about your plate more in depth in Chapter 3, but these components are vital to a healthy metabolism now.)

**Move your body every day!** The more you are active, the more active your metabolism! The more muscle you have, the more fuel your body needs to maintain the mass. Muscle burns ten times more calories than other tissue. One pound of body fat burns 5 calories per day compared to 1 pound of muscle that burns *50 calories per day!* Does strength training sound more attractive now? Your lean muscle mass is one of the most significant factors in your metabolic rate. Your body needs an abundance of energy to keep your muscle tissue muscle!

**Sleep.** The US Department of Health and Human services recommends adults need about seven to eight hours, teens need at least nine hours, children need ten to twelve hours, and babies need sixteen to eighteen hours of sleep every day. Not only is getting adequate sleep a necessity, it has a variety of health benefits:

- You will be less likely to get sick.

- You lower your risk of high blood pressure and diabetes.

- You boost your brainpower and your mood.

- You think more clearly and do better in school and at work.

**For Better Sleep (Lawrence Epstein, MD):**

- Keep a regular sleep/wake schedule.

- Develop a pre-sleep routine.

- Reserve the bedroom for sleep and intimacy.

- Practice daily exercise to burn off extra energy.

- Maintain a healthy diet.

- Do not drink to excess or smoke.

Circle the points you can work on to start sleeping better.

- You make better decisions and avoid injuries; sleepy drivers cause thousands of car crashes every year.

- *You will be more likely to maintain a healthy weight.*

## A Toxic Metabolism

The cells of your body are largely made up of what you feed them. Likewise, your metabolism functions from everything you eat. If you are consistently overeating sugar and toxins, your body is full of the chemicals it takes to process and break down the contaminations (as well as the toxins themselves). Toxins put stress on every organ in your body. For example, if you consistently ingest too much sodium, your heart must work extra hard to eliminate the extra salt from the body, stressing your heart. *Too much* of anything is tantamount to *not enough.*

> *I found that cleaning out my pantry of processed foods helped me prepare for a healthier lifestyle and it played an enormous role in not going backward with my eating habits.*
>
> GAO F.
> INFIT CLIENT

Not enough nourishment is just as damaging as overeating. We eat because we like the taste of food. Manufacturers know this. They study your preferences and base their careers on producing cheap, delicious food. Often this results in adding pernicious chemicals to your food to hyper-excite your taste buds.

Reading labels is an essential part of recognizing food as nourishment because, while chemical additives may excite your taste buds, they do not love and honor your DNA. On the contrary, chemical additives break down and destroy our DNA and put us at risk for a whole host of diseases.

When you shop, take the list below or the expanded list in the appendix. It may seem cumbersome to read every label in the store, *but I promise it is worth your time.* You will soon be able to recognize what you are looking for. You will feel better, look better, have more energy, and have fewer toxins in your body. And, the more aware of labels you are, the easier shopping gets. You will know which brands have clean ingredients and which brands go the cheaper, chemical, and processed route.

## Ingredients to Avoid (See Expanded List in Appendix)

### Harmful Preservatives

I say harmful because some forms of preserving food are not damaging. For example, if you put your grapes in the freezer, this will preserve them, but it will not harm the food in the process.

*Partially hydrogenated oil*—This is a harmful preservative that adds hydrogen to the oil at a high heat. According to the Mayo Clinic, this process of adding hydrogen to preserve the oil negatively throws off the balance of your cholesterol (LDL/HDL) among a long list of terrible health implications that we will tackle in Chapter 7. Have you ever seen a fast-food burger that was (purposefully) left out in the doctor's office for years *and it did not look any different then when it was bought?* Think about how it looks in your body. The substance does not effortlessly break down because of the massive amount of preservatives in the burger. No meat, cheese, or carbohydrate should be able to sit out in the open without decomposing. Avoid putting anything in your body that is pumped with embalming-like oil. I tell my clients to think about partially hydrogenated oils like liquid glue added to the oil. It sticks to your body and does *not* easily break down. Have you ever quit eating fast food for a period of time and then caved in and ate a fast-food cheeseburger and fries or some variety of fried food? That stomachache you got after eating was the food sitting in your stomach like a magnetic lump of glue, attracting bad bacteria. Ugh. It is no wonder we have so many stomach problems. Avoid preservatives and you will reduce your stomach complications.

*BHA and BHT*—Otherwise known as butylated hydroxyanisole and butylated hydroxytoluene. Similar to partially hydrogenated oils, these preservatives keep the last leftover perishable nutrients in highly processed oils in foods from going rancid. They do not belong in food because your body does not recognize the chemicals. Along with highly processed oils, unrecognizable chemicals are suggested to increase your chances of getting cancer.

*Sodium Benzoate, nitrates and nitrites, sulfates, potassium bromate*—Like all the chemicals above, they do not belong in your body, and they should be avoided as much as possible.

There are whole books dedicated to the harmful effects of preservatives in our foods. They key is to look for whole food recipes that you can prepare yourself and then preserve naturally. Limit your intake of packaged foods as meals and snacks. Balanced eating does not have to be all or nothing. Real plants and animal foods are not evil. The more we are mindful of what we put in our bodies, the better we will look and feel.

## Flavor Enhancers

*Artificial sweeteners, aspartame, and sucralose (Splenda®)*—The problem with artificial, zero-calorie sweeteners is not necessarily in the chemicals themselves, but in the damage they do to our intestines, brain, and hormones once they are in the body.

*Monosodium glutamate (MSG)*—This food additive has *no purpose* other than to enhance the flavor of food and get you addicted. MSG is found in some soy sauces, chips, frozen vegetable mixes, seasonings, soups, salad dressings, and packaged foods. MSG is a thyroid killer, a metabolic murderer, and a brain-sensory thief, an all-around thug. Need I say more? Read labels.

## Enriched Grains

This is one of the most misleading ingredients I have found on the market. The word *enriched* sounds like a promising description, right? I am sorry to disappoint, but in the context of grains, the "enriching" process leaves the product impoverished. Imagine taking your most precious *real* pearl necklace or bracelet and

In addition to body fat percentage testing, another accurate test for body composition is the *waist circumference measurement*. Take a tape measurement around the largest part of your belly button and record the number.

**Waist Circumference:**

For women, a healthy belly button circumference is under 35 inches and for men, under 40 inches.

**The C-Word**

I hesitate using the word cancer in this book because when used, it gives us permission to make a statement like "everything causes cancer these days." This statement is *not* true and allowing ourselves to believe this lie is fatal to our health. Not everything causes cancer.

Certain chemicals have been suggested to cause cancer. As we add more and more artificial chemicals, preservatives, colors, and flavor enhancers to foods, that list continues to grow.

### Cholesterol Truth

The myth about cholesterol is that it is all bad. The truth is that cholesterol is so important, your body makes approximately 1,000 milligrams per day! Scientific studies prove that dietary cholesterol has little effect on the cholesterol levels found in your blood.

Cholesterol is important in protecting your nerves, brain, and the walls of your intestines.

Elevated levels of cholesterol in the blood are linked to heart disease, *but dietary cholesterol is not the direct cause of heart disease.*

Plaque buildup and injury and narrowing of the blood vessels are mainly caused from:

- Inflammation
- Deep-fried food
- Partially hydrogenated oils
- Oxidized fats (heated oils)
- High blood glucose
- Lack of antioxidants and essential nutrients
- Stress hormones
- High blood pressure

ripping all the pearls off and throwing them away. Then, imagine cutting out pictures of pearls from paper and gluing them on the strand. You would look at the final product and say *something is wrong here.* This stripping of the original nutrients is the process that most grains experience in America. Whole kernels of wheat, rice, oat, cornmeal, or barley are all rich in fiber, B vitamins, iron, folate, calcium, phosphorus, zinc, and copper. These are nutrients that your body (and brain) desperately need to maintain balance for your health. When grains are processed, they are stripped of many of these nutrients and then bleached to create a color and texture that manufacturers want us to enjoy. The problem is that when manufacturers realize the end product is not much more than play dough, they enrich the grain much like the paper cut-out version of your pearls. Original nutrients such as fiber and B vitamins are thrown away in the refining process. B vitamins are mood boosters. When we consume enriched breads, muffins, bagels, and pasta, we are *not* receiving the natural form of this important vitamin that helps balance our brains and boost our moods. Fiber is another nutrient that is not adequately replaced in the enriching process. Fiber acts like a magnet, absorbing and eliminating toxins and improving the function of your colon. We need these natural nutrients, not from synthetic enriching, but from the real, whole foods!

## Artificial Colors

Pause. Any time you read the word *artificial*, think *do I want any artificial additive in my body?* The answer should be no, but some are necessary (like a life-saving drug) and some are not (like artificial colors). If you see the name of the color and a number in the ingredients, the color is artificial (yellow 5, for example). Imagine sticking a crayon up into your brain and trying to function. You would definitely have some attention challenges with yellow 5 in the middle of your cerebellum.

Look at a 2009 quote from Colombia University on mental health studies:

"This [tremendous effect] was similar to the effect size reported in an earlier meta-analysis conducted by researchers at Columbia University and Harvard University. Their analysis of fifteen trials evaluating the impact of artificial food coloring suggests that removing these agents from the diets of children with ADHD would be about 1/3 to 1/2 as effective as treatment with methylphenidate (Ritalin)."

This research is suggesting that *by cutting out artificial colors, children with ADHD will have 1/3 to 1/2 fewer symptoms!* This study should be a wakeup call for all of us. Artificial colors are not healthy for our brains. This is just one small piece of the brain puzzle. The article goes on to explain what is missing from our daily nutrient intake, Omega-3s and other essential vitamins and minerals, and how those too play a vital role in our (and our children's) mental health. In addition to brain problems, artificial colors have been linked to fatigue, allergic reactions, skin rashes, asthma, and headaches. *Be more aware of what you are putting in your body and how it affects your health*. You are not a victim. You have options. You can make a difference in how you (and your children) look and feel by taking the time to think about what goes in your (and their) mouth(s).

## Break It Down with Comparisons

Partially hydrogenated oil is comparable to glue.

*Look for this instead: virgin or extra virgin oils.*

Enriched flour is comparable to play dough.

*Look for this instead: whole grains as the first and only source of grain and at least 3 grams of fiber per serving (preferably sprouted grains when available for best nutrients and absorbability).*

Artificial additives are comparable to poison.

*Look for this instead: Food that is naturally colored and flavored with fruit or vegetables rather than artificially colored with coal tar and petroleum* (which are the real ingredients in most artificial colors).

## The Good News

Regardless of what you have been consuming or how long you have been consuming it, you can make small changes in what you eat that will have an immediate and lasting effect on the health of your body, mind, and soul. You were made for more than mediocre nutrition. You were made for more than working out once every January. *You were made for exceptional health.*

Recap—Start small. Make realistic, healthy changes starting with thinking about food as nourishment rather than fuel alone. Consistent small steps lead to a lifetime of wellness habits and a healthier you.

What did you eat for breakfast today?

Was it mostly empty fuel or did it also nourish your body?

_____

How soon after you ate did you become hungry again?

_____

### Body Composition

BMI stands for body mass index. It is measurement of an individual's body composition based on height and weight. For some, this tool is an accurate measure of health. However, for many individuals (especially those with high lean muscle mass), BMI is not the most accurate measurement available. This method is often used because it is quick and easy, not requiring anything more than a scale and a calculator. A healthy BMI range for men and women is between 18.5-24.9.

In addition to getting your BMI calculated, get your **body fat percentage** tested from a doctor or certified personal trainer and compare the results. A healthy body fat percentage range for women is between 14-29% and for men it is between 6-24%.

### Chew Your Food!

Problems arise in your digestive system when you have large pieces of unchewed food floating around. Take your time and chew your food slowly for optimal digestion!

### *What Is Considered a "Whole Food"?

A whole food is minimally processed, something you can pluck, harvest, fish, or hunt.

## Metabolism

Do you notice a connection between feeling sluggish and tired after making poor nutrition and fitness choices? Yes/No

Why?

_____

What choices are you making that negatively affect your metabolism?

_____

What do you do well to keep your metabolism healthy (refer to the five steps)?

_____

Keep practicing your metabolism boosting skills until they become habits and then move on to another skill to continue improving the efficiency of your metabolism. If *what* you are eating is healthy, your body will be burning food efficiently, and *if* you are in your calorie range to lose weight, your metabolism will begin to burn fat as fuel, rather than store it in all the wrong places.

**Tip from Your Trainer:** Presentation is powerful. If you or your children are regularly consuming high-sugar cereal full of artificial color, find a low-sugar, non-artificially sweetened yogurt they enjoy and add a few colorful fruits like blueberries, sliced strawberries, and sliced mango. Invest in some visually pleasing, *small* dessert bowls (Goodwill is a great place to find colorful, inexpensive dessert bowls). Slice up extra strawberries and mango for a snack to use in tomorrow's fruit and yogurt parfait. Lemon juice on the fruit will prevent it from browning. The prep takes slightly longer than pouring cereal and milk, yet the results affect your and your family's brain health—minimal food preparation goes a long way!

## Practice

Continue recognizing *why* you eat. Are you hungry? Are you thirsty? Are you bored? Are you addicted? Are you sad? Is your body lacking a nutrient? When you recognize the signals of your body, you are able to make better decisions. Consistent healthy decisions lead to better health (and usually weight loss if that is one of your goals).

Ninety-five percent of your food should be for nourishment. Treats should be saved for rare and special occasions like birthdays and graduations. Before you reach for your next meal or snack, ask yourself, *will this food or beverage nourish my body or is it simply providing fuel or pleasure?*

Read labels. If you do not have time to read every single label (I recommend eventually getting in this habit), start by reading all your breakfast labels and avoid added sugar, artificial colors, flavors, and preservatives. Look for whole grains and whole foods for breakfast instead of colorful, sugary cereal (remember that study on artificial colors and children). Initially, your family may not be happy with your nutritional changes, but consider that any change is challenging at first. I promise the payoff is worth the effort.

## S2L

We learn best when we share information with others. Discuss how to increase the health and efficiency of your metabolism with someone. Review one ingredient to avoid when reading labels. If you can repeat the facts, you can recall the facts. The more you understand what it takes to have abundant energy and a high-functioning metabolism, the more you will be able to assess how to improve your health on days when you are sluggish and tired.

Who are you going to discuss the metabolism with?

_____

What are you going to teach them?

_____

Which food additive are you going to teach them about?

_____

Do not skip the S2L sections—they work!

## Sea Salt Cocoa-Covered Cashews (or Almonds)

*Ashley's Favorite Dessert Recipe (Serves 1)*

This recipe is easy, delicious, and healthy—it contains zero grams of refined sugar!

### Ingredients

- 1 tablespoon almond butter
- 1 teaspoon raw honey (locally sourced honey is best)
- 1 tablespoon raw cocoa powder
- 1 tablespoon raw coconut oil
- 1/4 teaspoon sea salt or mineral salt (use only a small pinch)
- 1/8 cup raw cashews or almonds

### Directions

In a small saucepan, heat almond butter and coconut oil on low until melted. Remove from heat. Add honey, cocoa powder, and salt, mixing well. Sprinkle the cashews or almonds in the mixture and enjoy! You can eat this treat with a spoon or dip in your favorite fruit. If you want to make the mixture into a homemade protein and fiber bar, scoop the mixture onto wax paper and let it cool in the fridge.

*Calories: 270*

# InFIT Workout 2

First time (set) through: Warm up: Go through all of the exercises slowly, 15-20 repetitions each, with no resistance (no weight), 5-10 minutes. Second set: Perform the exercises one at a time, with resistance when appropriate, starting with one lower body exercise, one upper body exercise, and one core exercise with minimal rest in between. Perform all nine exercises and repeat as your fitness goals and time permit! Remember to drink water during your workout and stretch tight muscles.

## Lower Body

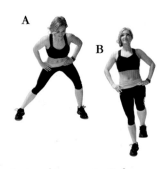

**Lateral Lunge to Balance**

|  | Set 1 | Set 2 |
|---|---|---|
| Weight |  |  |
| Reps |  |  |

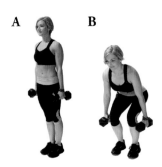

**DB Squat**

|  | Set 1 | Set 2 |
|---|---|---|
| Weight |  |  |
| Reps |  |  |

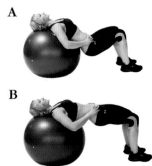

**SB Bridge–Double Leg**

|  | Set 1 | Set 2 |
|---|---|---|
| Weight |  |  |
| Reps |  |  |

## Upper Body

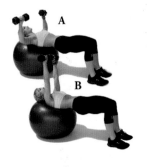

**DB SB Chest Press**

|  | Set 1 | Set 2 |
|---|---|---|
| Weight |  |  |
| Reps |  |  |

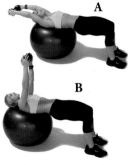

**DB SB Lat Extension**

|  | Set 1 | Set 2 |
|---|---|---|
| Weight |  |  |
| Reps |  |  |

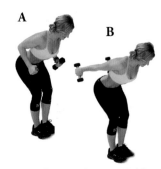

**DB Bent Over Triceps Kickback**

|  | Set 1 | Set 2 |
|---|---|---|
| Weight |  |  |
| Reps |  |  |

## Core

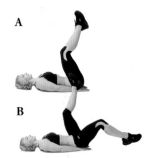

**Scissor Kick–Bent Legs**

|  | Set 1 | Set 2 |
|---|---|---|
| Weight |  |  |
| Reps |  |  |

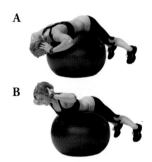

**SB Back Extension**

|  | Set 1 | Set 2 |
|---|---|---|
| Weight |  |  |
| Reps |  |  |

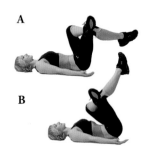

**Cross-Leg Reverse Crunch**

|  | Set 1 | Set 2 |
|---|---|---|
| Weight |  |  |
| Reps |  |  |

# InFIT Workout 2–Option II

Several exercises fall into more than one category. InFIT Workout 1 categorizes a bridge as a core exercise because your core muscles do the work, not your limbs (arms and legs). This workout also classifies a bridge as a lower body exercise, because your glutes are considered part of your lower body. One goal in fitness efficiency is to perfect basic exercises and then combine the exercises to make them more efficient. Full-body exercise equals efficiency and maximum tone. Perform all nine exercises and repeat as your fitness goals and time permit! Remember to drink water during your workout and stretch tight muscles.

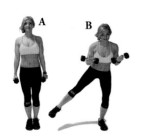

**DB Lateral Lunge to Balance with Biceps Curl**

|  | Set 1 | Set 2 |
|---|---|---|
| Weight |  |  |
| Reps |  |  |

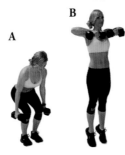

**DB Squat with Upright Row to Toes**

|  | Set 1 | Set 2 |
|---|---|---|
| Weight |  |  |
| Reps |  |  |

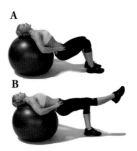

**SB Bridge–Single Leg**

|  | Set 1 | Set 2 |
|---|---|---|
| Weight |  |  |
| Reps |  |  |

*Lower Body*

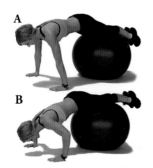

**SB Pushup**

|  | Set 1 | Set 2 |
|---|---|---|
| Weight |  |  |
| Reps |  |  |

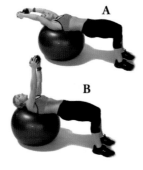

**DB SB Lat Extension–Heavier Weight**

|  | Set 1 | Set 2 |
|---|---|---|
| Weight |  |  |
| Reps |  |  |

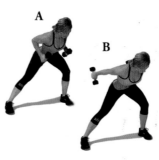

**DB ISO Lateral Lunge Triceps Kickback**

|  | Set 1 | Set 2 |
|---|---|---|
| Weight |  |  |
| Reps |  |  |

*Upper Body*

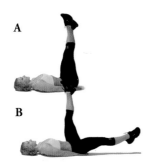

**Scissor Kick–Straight Leg**

|  | Set 1 | Set 2 |
|---|---|---|
| Weight |  |  |
| Reps |  |  |

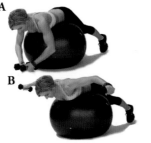

**DB SB Back Extension with Reverse Fly**

|  | Set 1 | Set 2 |
|---|---|---|
| Weight |  |  |
| Reps |  |  |

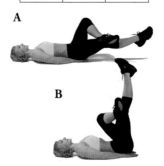

**Cross-Leg Reverse Crunch– Straight Leg**

|  | Set 1 | Set 2 |
|---|---|---|
| Weight |  |  |
| Reps |  |  |

*Core*

## Review Your Map—Chapter Reflection

Use this road map as a weekly check-in to measure your goals and progress. Fill in the blank spaces at the bottom of the chart to create your own goals. The more often you check in with yourself, the more often you will bring health to the front of your mind, creating intention and success.

| | GOAL | MON | TUE | WED | THU | FRI | SAT | SUN |
|---|---|---|---|---|---|---|---|---|
| | | Actual | Actual | Actual | Actual | Actual | Actual | Actual |
| **Servings of produce (Ch 5)** | | | | | | | | |
| **Water in ounces** | | | | | | | | |
| **Hours of sleep (Ch 2)** | | | | | | | | |
| **Minutes of exercise** | | | | | | | | |
| **Weight** | | | | | | | | |
| **Amount of meals/ snacks per day (Ch 3)** | | | | | | | | |
| **Calories** | | | | | | | | |
| **Number of simple carbs (Ch 6)** | | | | | | | | |
| **Body fat % (optional)** | | | | | | | | |
| **Bowel movements (Ch 8)** | | | | | | | | |
| **Add your own below** | | | | | | | | |
| | | | | | | | | |
| | | | | | | | | |
| | | | | | | | | |

Did you achieve most of your goals? _____ Why? _____

What is your plan for the next week to either stay on your original course or modify based on this week's review?

How do you feel about your progress thus far?

# LIVING AFFIRMATION
WELLNESS FOR YOUR SOUL

## Motives

Then the Lord God called to Adam and said to him, "Where are you?" So he said, "I heard Your voice in the garden, and I was afraid because I was naked; and I hid myself." Genesis 3:9-10

Why do you make the choices you do? Why do I make the choices I do? Asking that question allowed the secrets of my heart to be revealed. I used to be motivated by the belief that I had to grab every opportunity that appealed to me. But I never checked back with God, believing I alone had to make my life successful.

However, just as God asked Adam, God asks you and me, "Where are you?"

*Where could we possibly try to hide in front of God? Why do we search for fulfillment in other places, such as food?*

Perhaps reading through Chapter 2, you started to realize that food has become more to you than just fuel and nourishment. Maybe food has become a crutch, an addiction, an excuse, or a substitute.

Maybe you have made food choices based on the desire to be satisfied, to be comforted, or to gain something meaningful—other than your ideal weight. Maybe your scale or your health testifies that something in your relationship with food is not in order.

God is jealously interested to be everything to you and does not to want share top priority with anyone or anything. If food has been more than fuel and nourishment in your life, be transparent with God and share your heart. Tell God what you need. God will meet you where you are.

Be blessed abundantly! ~ *Christina Zaczkowski*, MA, CPT

## *Reflection*

_____

_____

_____

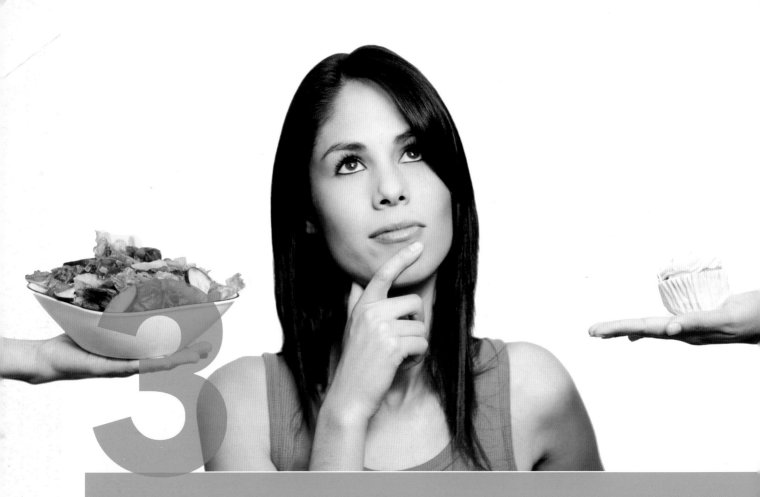

# WHAT SHOULD YOU EAT?

### Principle Questions:

1. Whose health are you putting before your own? How is this helping or harming you? What is the long-term effect of this choice?

2. What should your plate look like at each meal?

3. Do you really need to eat something from each food group every day?

4. What foods should you avoid and what healthy choices can you make instead?

5. What does successful meal planning look like?

Most of us take the time to feed our children, nieces and nephews, and/or grandchildren healthy food. "Eat your vegetables," we say to our little ones. While we are slicing up fresh strawberries for others, how about setting aside a serving for ourselves? While we are picking out a veggie that our children (or spouses) will like, could we select one that we like also? Most of us have put ourselves last in the household food chain. While it may look honorable on the surface to sacrifice yourself, you are not doing your health any favors. When our health suffers, when our depression rises, and our bodies fail us, *who can we help*? Who can we serve when we have no more energy? If we neglect our responsibility for our own wellness, the cost will probably be paid by the next generation.

We are an overgrained, oversugared, oversodiumed, undernourished society. Most people in industrial nations no longer perform physical jobs that require high-carbohydrate, high-energy meals. We just do not need as many carbs or calories. So what should you eat? Do you know what percentage of calories should come from carbohydrates, fats, and proteins? Does this change if you are trying to lose weight? What does this look like practically in everyday life? We will begin to unveil many rewarding answers in this chapter!

Do you remember the food pyramid that was introduced in 1991, with a thick base of a whopping six to eleven servings of grains recommended per day? Obviously influenced by a few government subsidized grain farmers in the '80s, this recommendation was *far off balance* for a society moving away from physically active jobs. Can you imagine eating eleven slices of bread or eleven cups of pasta per day? If you think pasta goes to your hips now . . . imagine following the old plan! The scary part is that although the recommendations have changed, *most of us are still consuming too many grains per day*. And the grains are now stripped of their nutritional value, turning into sugar almost instantly in our bodies, creating an addictive, fat-storing cycle.

Measure and count how many servings of grains you are eating for three days and record it here:

Day 1 _____

Day 2 _____

Day 3 _____

What did you discover?

_____

When you measured serving sizes (especially foods like cereal and pasta), were you surprised? Yes/No

What are your favorite foods?

When balancing the food groups on your plate, what do you think you will struggle with?

What changes will be easy for you to create a healthier plate?

# Breaking the Fat-Storing Cycle

This is the government's current recommendation from the USDA's MyPlate. It is overly simplistic and lacks the necessity of water, healthy fats and oils, and the importance of whole grains.

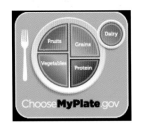

For individuals who are physically active during the day or those who exercise on a regular basis, the Harvard School of Public Health model offers a more promising plan. Because you are unique, your needs are different from the needs of others. Based on more than a decade of experience and repeated long-term client success stories, I recommend modeling your meals after the Harvard Healthy Eating Plate and adjusting your plan as you learn more about your body.

**Tip from Your Trainer:** Your metabolism usually burns more efficiently toward the beginning of the day. Eat fruit before dinner for optimal sugar burning.

Remember: *Optimal nutrition is not about, "is this food good or bad." Optimal nutrition is about choosing your best option in the given circumstance.* Sometimes, the best thing we can do on the road is to stop at a gas station for a meal or snack. Instead of grabbing a hot dog for lunch, how about:

- Cheese stick (protein)
- Almonds (fats)
- Apple or banana (fruits)
- Raw vegetable medley (vegetables)
- Bottle of water (or filtered tap water)

You can get that lunch for less than five dollars at most gas stations—way more healthy than fast food, and it is affordable.

## Let's Break It Down

### Produce

Half your plate for every meal and snack should be fruits and/or vegetables. Unlike the MyPlate model, the Harvard plate shows how much more produce should come from vegetables rather than fruit. Fruit is healthy and packed with vitamins, but it is also higher in sugar (fructose), which can cause an inflammatory response in the body

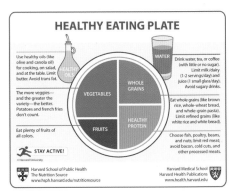

Copyright © 2011 Harvard University. For more information about The Healthy Eating Plate, please see The Nutrition Source, Department of Nutrition, Harvard School of Public Health, www.thenutritionsource.org and Harvard Health Publications, health.harvard.edu.

when too much is consumed. Sugar makes weight loss more challenging because it raises insulin levels. Insulin crushes hormones that allow your body to use fat as the main source of fuel. We will look at the necessity of pairing produce with healthy fat, protein, and fiber in Chapters 5, 6, and 7.

### Grains

Based on the role of grains and protein, my experience has been that individuals whose goal is to lose weight experience more success when they emphasize healthy fats and protein over grains and simple carbohydrates. This does not mean eliminating all grains from your diet. Emphasizing weight loss means looking at your plate and occasionally choosing healthy protein and fat over grains and often choosing veggies (complex carbohydrates) over simple carbohydrates. We will talk extensively about the reason for this in the carbohydrate and protein chapters, but let's tackle the basics. A few simple carbohydrates include:

- White bread
- White rice
- Enriched/white pasta
- Soda
- Highly processed foods
- Muffins
- Bagels
- Crackers*

These foods have little to no nutritional value. They act as refined sugar in your body. They absorb quickly into the blood stream and leave you feeling hungry soon after eating. Also, they contain little or no fiber to aid in digestion. If your grains are not 100% whole, you may as well be eating play dough.

## Protein

Unlike simple carbohydrates, protein takes longer to break down, leaving you with an extended sense of fullness. Additionally, protein is responsible for rebuilding and repairing damaged cells. Not all protein is created equal; according to the Harvard School of Public Health, poultry, fish, beans, and nuts are the best sources of protein. If you are very physically active, you will need more protein than what is recommended for the average person. We will get into specifics in Chapter 4.

## Dietary Fats

In the MyPlate model, healthy oils are neglected all together. Healthy fats and oils play a vital role in nutrient absorption, digestion, and brain health, and they should be incorporated into *every* meal and snack. Approximately 35-45% of your daily calories should come from healthy dietary fat sources. We will get into the details in Chapter 6.

## What Should You Eat?

Based off of the Harvard Healthy Eating Plate, the charts below offer ideas for foods to avoid and healthier alternatives to try instead. *Remember, optimal health is not about "is this food good or bad." Optimal health is about what is your best choice in this circumstance!* Meal planning helps you make better choices. Meal planning puts you in the driver seat during your road trip, rather than being trapped in your trunk! Let's look at examples of foods and snacks we should avoid, what to eat instead, and then plan out our *own* meals for the next seven days. Use the circular meal plans (yes, they look like "Mickey Mouse") in the appendix for your meals and snacks. Make copies for yourself so you can repeat the process!

**\*Reminder from Chapter 2:**

Look for food that will *nourish* you, not just provide fuel.

What healthy changes can you make right now to your regular breakfast routine?

Which lunch ideas appeal to you?

What food choices will you struggle with?

What food choices will be easy for you?

*"By failing to prepare, you are preparing to fail."*
BENJAMIN FRANKLIN

# Breakfast Ideas

| Avoid | Try Instead |
|---|---|
| Cereal and milk | 1/2 cup 2% yogurt, 1/4 cup fruit, 1/8 cup low sugar (10 grams or less) granola |
| Bagel and cream cheese | 2 scrambled eggs and 1 ounce natural cheese |
| White toast and margarine | 100% whole-grain sprouted toast and 1 tablespoon butter and 1/2 cup sliced strawberries on side |
| Doughnut and coffee | Smoothie: 1 banana, 1 tablespoon almond butter, and 1 cup unsweetened almond milk |
| Pancakes and bacon | 2 hardboiled eggs and 6 ounces orange juice (or try a whole orange instead for more fiber) |

# Lunch Ideas

| Avoid | Try Instead |
|---|---|
| Fast-food burger | Fast-food salad—dressing on the side |
| Frozen pasta meal | Frozen veggies, rice, chicken, and cheese (leftover from dinner—see below) |
| Sandwich with packaged meat | Salad with protein, nuts, veggies, and cheese |
| Fried food or fried appetizers | Chicken skewers, beef tips, and/or salsa with celery |
| Canned soup high in sodium | Homemade soup with veggies and protein or canned soup with less sodium |

# Dinner Ideas

| Avoid | Try Instead |
|---|---|
| Pasta or potatoes as the main course | Try fresh or lightly steamed veggies as the main course—*get creative with new spices* |
| Fried food | Try taking a baked, steamed, or grilled approach to your traditional fried recipes |
| Packaged foods for most dinners | Try to make enough dinner to last one or two days for leftovers |
| Highly processed meat and veggies (think frozen dinners) | Look for meat without nitrites, nitrates, and other additives. Add wild-caught fish one to two times per week. |
| High sugar desserts | Try 2% plain yogurt with honey and fruit for dessert |

Finally, the most challenging for most Americans . . . *snacks*. Snacks can make or break your food budget, your meal plan, and your scale.

## Snack Attack!

| Avoid | Try Instead |
|---|---|
| Protein bars with more than 10 grams of sugar per serving | Lettuce wrap with protein and natural sweet chili sauce |
| Corn chips or pretzels and dip | Veggies and one serving of hummus or salsa |
| Candy bar | 1 fruit and 1/2 cup 2% cottage cheese |
| Fast-food mini meal | 1 serving of nuts, no-sugar added dried fruit, and 7 or 8 dark chocolate chips (for chocolate lovers) |
| Enriched crackers and artificial cheese dip | 100% whole-grain crackers and 1 ounce of cheese |

Make a point to go to the fridge (where you have fresh produce) for a snack rather than the pantry (where you have packaged goods). Be sure to stock up on fresh, frozen, canned, and dehydrated produce and protein so you are not stuck with the junk when you run out of fresh, whole foods.

Now, let's do some meal planning with the foods you love!

## Common Sense Meal Planning

What will you eat for breakfast tomorrow and for the rest of the week?

Day 1 _____

Day 2 _____

Day 3 _____

Day 4 _____

Day 5 _____

Day 6 _____

Day 7 _____

### How Often Should You Eat Dessert?

Some people think dessert should accompany every meal. This mindset keeps us thinking that dessert is a norm. Dessert that includes added sugar should be a rare treat; at most, one serving per day, and dessert should fit within a healthy portion size and calorie guidelines.

I went all the way to Day 7 because as we learned in Chapters 1 and 2, a five days on, two days off approach is *not* the most successful way to be healthy or lose weight long-term. Health is not a diet. *Living Wellness* is not a program you try for a while and then fail. *Living Wellness* is a lifestyle. Health is a choice. There will be days that are better than others. You will deviate from your meal plan. But the point is you have a plan and you will make your choices. The more consistently you *choose health* over convenience, peer pressure, or lack of motivation, the more quickly your pallet will change and your body will begin to *crave* the foods it was made for. You will then struggle less to make better decisions. If one of your health goals is

*Planning weekly meal calendars and sticking them on our fridge helps our entire family stay on track. It also encourages healthier eating when going out to eat might seem like the "easy" option.*

MELISSA H.
INFIT INSTRUCTOR AND
ALLÉE CEO

## Out of Sight . . .

Keep junk food out of the house! "Out of sight, out of mind" is an effective motto. If ice cream is your weakness, *do not* buy it. If you eat a whole bag of chips in one sitting, avoid buying chips until you have established discipline—or do not buy them at all. Save yourself money and buy a good pair of running shoes instead.

to lose 1 pound of body fat per week, what calorie deficit do you need in seven days? If you said *3,500 calories, you are correct!* Now, let's say you are spot on for five days, reducing 500 calories per day from a combination of nutrition and exercise; you are so close you can almost feel your jeans getting looser. As a reward, you decide to take a day off. You will not count calories, but you will be careful not to go crazy; perhaps you will just allow yourself to revert back to some old habits:

- Cereal with milk and coffee with cream for breakfast

- Chips and salsa for snack

- Chipotle burrito for lunch (you skipped the cheese to save some calories)

- Energy bar and soda for snack

- Tator-tot hotdish and mashed potatoes for dinner

Look familiar? It does to me. I used to eat like this far too often! I thought I was healthy by skipping the cheese on my burrito. I did not know any better. This meal plan is around *2,700 calories—for one day!* Another day like this and the whole week's plan has been tanked and reversed. *Remember, you are not on a diet.* You can choose to eat whatever you want, whenever you want . . . but you were created for more than mediocre health. You were created for exceptional health, waking up feeling good every day, and making informed decisions one day at a time toward this goal.

**Tip from Your Trainer:** When eating out at a fast-food or sit-down restaurant, think about what you will eat before you get there. You know you probably will not resist temptation when you are hungry and the tantalizing smell of food is in the air. Make your choice based on something you would not necessarily make at home, like grilled poultry, fish, or a fancy salad. Ask for a box before you get your food and take half home for lunch the next day or split the meal with a friend. Every time you make a healthy choice when eating out, you will feel good about your decision and it will be easier to make the next decision a healthy one.

Let's continue looking at your meal planning using circles. Refer back to the Harvard Healthy Eating Plate for specific guidelines. Complete one plate per meal. See the appendix for a worksheet on meal planning and grocery shopping for the entire week. Make copies for personal use.

What will one lunch plan look like this week?

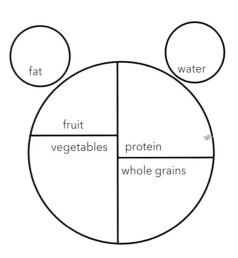

What will one dinner plan look like this week?

What will one snack look like this week?

## Keys: Balance and Variety

Do you have a better sense of what to eat now? If not, go back to the beginning of this chapter and review. The keys of successful meal planning are in a balance of food groups and a variety of nutrients. If you start your journey eating similar foods for every meal, do not stress out. Once you develop consistent routines, you can start replacing your regular protein for a new protein, your regular veggies for a new veggie, and your regular grains for new grains (and maybe eventually seeds!) Continue practicing meal planning: It will soon become a healthy habit.

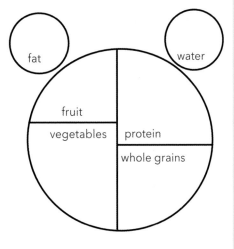

fat

water

fruit

vegetables  protein

whole grains

## Practice

Track your progress. Continue writing in your wellness journal and choose food for fuel *and* nourishment.

Build variety. When grocery shopping, pick up a variety of fresh, frozen, canned, and dried produce and protein to avoid turning to junk food when you run out of fresh, whole foods or for convenience.

Think ahead. Plan out your meals a couple of days in advance and bring your plan to the store. Have a backup plan of healthier fast-food options and pack nutritious snacks in your car for "emergencies."

## S2L

Take this week to teach someone about MyPlate or the Healthy Food Plate. Discuss your meal planning ideas with someone.

What did you learn from sharing meal planning ideas?

Discuss the government's MyPlate and Harvard Healthy Food Plate.

Which model fits your life better?

*Just because you do not have much to choose from does not mean you cannot choose wisely.*

JAY SHEARER, JJ SHEARER COMPANY CEO

What groceries do you need in order to make this meal plan happen? See the full grocery shopping list in the appendix.

*When grocery shopping, remember to buy a variety of fresh, frozen, canned, and dried or dehydrated produce and meat so you can stay focused when you run out of fresh, whole foods.*

### Pack a Cooler

When I am out of my house for several hours with my two children, I have them pack their own snacks and meals for the day. We put snacks and meals in a small cooler and/or grocery bag, with foods and beverages like:

- Cheese sticks
- Yogurt (we have even made our own frozen yogurt tubes)
- Raw nuts
- Bag of veggies with natural hummus
- Several pieces of washed fruit
- Bottled water

# InFIT Workout 3

First time (set) through: Warm up: Go through all of the exercises slowly, 15-20 repetitions each, with no resistance (no weight), 5-10 minutes. Second set: Perform the exercises one at a time, with resistance when appropriate, starting with one lower body exercise, one upper body exercise, and one core exercise with minimal rest in between. Perform all nine exercises and repeat as your fitness goals and time permit! Remember to drink water during your workout and stretch tight muscles!

**Lower Body**

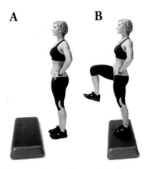

### Front Step-Up to Balance

|         | Set 1 | Set 2 |
|---------|-------|-------|
| Weight  |       |       |
| Reps    |       |       |

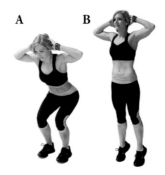

### Prisoner Squat to Toes

|         | Set 1 | Set 2 |
|---------|-------|-------|
| Weight  |       |       |
| Reps    |       |       |

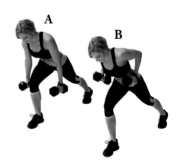

### DB Lunge with Row

|         | Set 1 | Set 2 |
|---------|-------|-------|
| Weight  |       |       |
| Reps    |       |       |

**Upper Body**

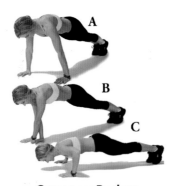

### Crossover Pushup

|         | Set 1 | Set 2 |
|---------|-------|-------|
| Weight  |       |       |
| Reps    |       |       |

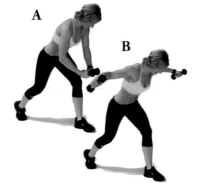

### DB Lunge Reverse Fly

|         | Set 1 | Set 2 |
|---------|-------|-------|
| Weight  |       |       |
| Reps    |       |       |

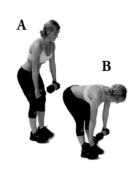

### DB Deadlift

|         | Set 1 | Set 2 |
|---------|-------|-------|
| Weight  |       |       |
| Reps    |       |       |

**Core**

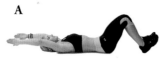
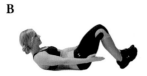

### Pilates Half Roll Up

|         | Set 1 | Set 2 |
|---------|-------|-------|
| Weight  |       |       |
| Reps    |       |       |

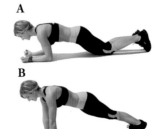

### Knees Plank to Pushup

|         | Set 1 | Set 2 |
|---------|-------|-------|
| Weight  |       |       |
| Reps    |       |       |

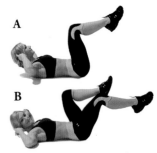

### Supine Bicycle

|         | Set 1 | Set 2 |
|---------|-------|-------|
| Weight  |       |       |
| Reps    |       |       |

# InFIT Workout 3—Option II

In InFIT Workout 3, Option II, we are still in the Stabilization Endurance Level, so remember: If you can perform more than 20 reps, increase your resistance. Perform all nine exercises and repeat as your fitness goals and time permit! Remember to drink water during your workout and stretch tight muscles!

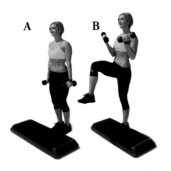

**Front Step-Up to Balance with Biceps Curl**

|         | Set 1 | Set 2 |
|---------|-------|-------|
| Weight  |       |       |
| Reps    |       |       |

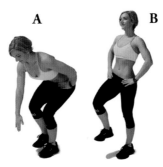

**Single Leg Squat Touchdown**

|         | Set 1 | Set 2 |
|---------|-------|-------|
| Weight  |       |       |
| Reps    |       |       |

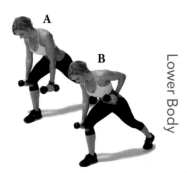

**Lunge with ALT Arm Row**

|         | Set 1 | Set 2 |
|---------|-------|-------|
| Weight  |       |       |
| Reps    |       |       |

Lower Body

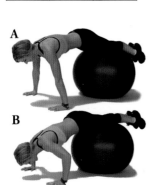

**SB Pushup**

|         | Set 1 | Set 2 |
|---------|-------|-------|
| Weight  |       |       |
| Reps    |       |       |

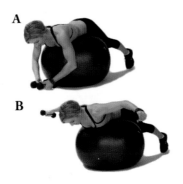

**DB SB Reverse Fly**

|         | Set 1 | Set 2 |
|---------|-------|-------|
| Weight  |       |       |
| Reps    |       |       |

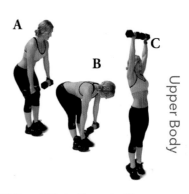

**DB Deadlift to Press to Toes**

|         | Set 1 | Set 2 |
|---------|-------|-------|
| Weight  |       |       |
| Reps    |       |       |

Upper Body

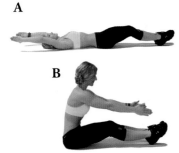

**Pilates Full Body Roll Up**

|         | Set 1 | Set 2 |
|---------|-------|-------|
| Weight  |       |       |
| Reps    |       |       |

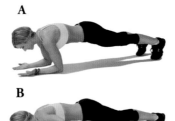

**Full Body Plank to Pushup**

|         | Set 1 | Set 2 |
|---------|-------|-------|
| Weight  |       |       |
| Reps    |       |       |

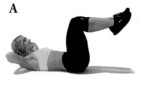
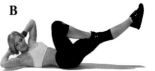

**Supine Bicycle–Straight Legs**

|         | Set 1 | Set 2 |
|---------|-------|-------|
| Weight  |       |       |
| Reps    |       |       |

Core

# ROAD MAP TO **SUCCESS**

## Review Your Map—Chapter Reflection

Use this road map as a weekly check-in to measure your goals and progress. Fill in the blank spaces at the bottom of the chart to create your own goals. The more often you check in with yourself, the more often you will bring health to the front of your mind, creating intention and success.

| | GOAL | MON Actual | TUE Actual | WED Actual | THU Actual | FRI Actual | SAT Actual | SUN Actual |
|---|---|---|---|---|---|---|---|---|
| **Servings of produce (Ch 5)** | | | | | | | | |
| **Water in ounces** | | | | | | | | |
| **Hours of sleep (Ch 2)** | | | | | | | | |
| **Minutes of exercise** | | | | | | | | |
| **Weight** | | | | | | | | |
| **Amount of meals/ snacks per day (Ch 3)** | | | | | | | | |
| **Calories** | | | | | | | | |
| **Number of simple carbs (Ch 6)** | | | | | | | | |
| **Body fat % (optional)** | | | | | | | | |
| **Bowel movements (Ch 8)** | | | | | | | | |
| **Add your own below** | | | | | | | | |
| | | | | | | | | |
| | | | | | | | | |
| | | | | | | | | |

Did you achieve most of your goals? _____ Why? _____

What is your plan for the next week to either stay on your original course or modify based on this week's review?

How do you feel about your progress thus far?

# LIVING AFFIRMATION
WELLNESS FOR YOUR SOUL

## Weary Worriers

Therefore I say to you, do not worry about your life, what you will eat or what you will drink; nor about your body, what you will put on. Is not life more than food and the body more than clothing? Matthew 6:25

We could justify our lack of knowledge about nutrition with the scripture verse from Matthew 6. We could say, Jesus tells me not to worry about what I eat, so I will not! However, back in the Garden of Eden, food choices were so simple; everything God intended us to eat was there, growing on trees, in the earth, or in the waters. The important question from Chapter 3 of "What should I eat?" is answered in abundance through the gifts of nature's food, not in processing factories or fast-food restaurants.

A vital part of physical life is food. Jesus tells us not to worry. *Does this mean we should eat whatever we want and not worry about the consequences?* No, we have the opportunity to make life-giving nutrition choices.

Just as God takes care of birds and flowers (see Matthew 6), God takes care of us. This promise of providence does not mean that we neglect our responsibilities in life because God will hand us a loaf of bread. As you live a life of dependence on God, you will find that God provides for all your needs, including what to eat.

So, next time you eat, be joyful instead of concerned. Give thanks to God for your healthy, nourishing food.

Be blessed abundantly! ~ *Christina Zaczkowski*, MA, CPT

## *Reflection*

_____

_____

_____

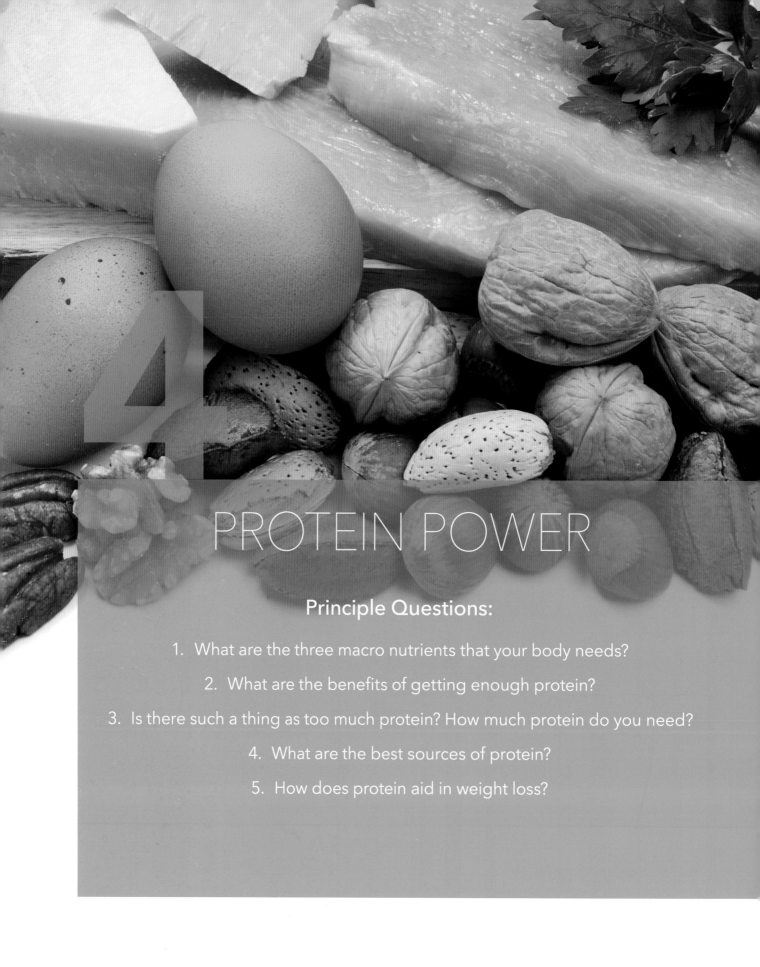

# PROTEIN POWER

## Principle Questions:

1. What are the three macro nutrients that your body needs?

2. What are the benefits of getting enough protein?

3. Is there such a thing as too much protein? How much protein do you need?

4. What are the best sources of protein?

5. How does protein aid in weight loss?

Protein has been a hot topic on the weight management stage since the Atkins diet. What is the big deal with protein? The three macro nutrients your body needs are protein, carbohydrates, and fat. Each one has unique properties and nutritious benefits. However, like all foods and beverages, consuming a balance of food groups and a variety of nutrients is vital to exceptional health. A lack of protein causes malnourishment, atrophy or muscle loss, failure to grow, weakened immune system, and weakened vital organs (the heart and respiratory system).

Likewise, getting too much protein without adequate water intake may have health risks as well. Breaking down and absorbing protein creates more waste than carbohydrates or fat, so if you are not consuming enough water, the process of eliminating the excess waste from your body may stress your liver or kidneys.

Two fundamentals to proper protein digestion include:

1. Eat enough quality and variety of protein.

2. Drink at least half of your ideal body weight in ounces every day.

## Protein:

- Rebuilds and repairs damaged cells resulting from the environment, working out, and illness

- Uses more calories to process, break down, and digest food over fat or carbohydrates. Example: It takes more energy to crush rock than to crush play dough. Your body uses more energy to digest protein, creating more of a calorie deficit.

## How Much Protein Is Just Right?

I hope you are not getting sick of this answer: *It varies from person to person*. Generally speaking, an adult should consume a minimum of 0.8 grams of protein per kilogram of body weight, which is about 8 grams of protein for every 20 pounds of body weight. For children, a minimum recommendation of protein is broken down by age:

## Recommended Dietary Allowance of Protein for Children

*Age Groups Grams of Protein Needed Per Day*

| | |
|---|---|
| Children ages 1-3 | **13** |
| Children ages 4-8 | **19** |
| Children ages 9-13 | **34** |
| Girls ages 14-18 | **46** |
| Boys ages 14-18 | **52** |

Use this area as a scratch pad for math calculations.

*"Do not let your fire go out, spark by irreplaceable spark in the hopeless swamps of the not-quite, the not-yet, and the not-at-all. Do not let the hero in your soul perish in lonely frustration for the life you deserved and have never been able to reach. The world you desire can be won. It exists . . . it is real . . . it is possible . . . it's yours."*

AYN RAND

## Getting Personal

What is the daily minimum recommendation of protein based on your weight? (Divide your body weight by 20 and then multiply that by 8 = _____ grams)

If you are an adult, use the recommendation based on your weight. If you are equating for a child, use the recommendation based on his or her age.

I do not count grams of protein for my children. Because they consume a variety of protein at every meal and snack, they receive adequate amounts. However, if you have a picky eater or a child with food sensitivities, you may want to count grams for a few days to ensure adequate amounts. If you realize your child is not consuming enough protein, try to increase their intake naturally. If your child(ren) are still not consuming enough, talk to your health care provider about your options for increasing protein intake with a supplement or shake.

If you work out several hours per week, you may need more protein to maintain, rebuild, and repair muscle and cell damage, which is a natural and healthy product of exercise. Muscle breakdown and repair allows our muscles to grow stronger. Be sure to check with your doctor before altering your nutrition beyond what is recommended.

Your body is better able to absorb protein at certain times during the day. Within one hour after your workout is the best time to consume one serving of protein with one serving of a complex carbohydrate. Let's look at some examples of post-exercise meals and snacks for optimal protein absorption.

## Good Sources of Protein

- Preservative-free meat, free-range poultry, and fish (wild-caught when available)

- Legumes (dry beans and peas)

- Eggs (from free-range, organic-fed chickens when available)

- Nuts and seeds (raw or sprouted is better than baked or roasted)

- Milk and milk products (from organic, grass-fed animals when available)

- 100% whole grains, some vegetables, and some fruits (all of these provide only small amounts of protein relative to animal sources)

These protein sources are also ideal as a part of every meal and snack.

## Do You Need a Protein Supplement, Powder, or Shake?

It is possible to get enough protein through dietary intake. Most individuals get more than enough protein per day. However, if you are not consuming enough protein (usually if you are getting protein from only vegetable sources), it is important to look for a supplement or shake with the following components.

What are your favorite sources of protein?

**Weight Management Benefits**

Protein satisfies, keeps you full longer, and uses more energy to digest than other fuel sources.

| Avoid | Look for instead |
|---|---|
| Hydrolyzed collagen or amino acid (incomplete proteins) | Egg white, whey, or casein |
| More than 5 grams of sugar per serving | 5 grams of sugar per serving or less |
| High levels of heavy metals | Low levels of heavy metals (check for arsenic, lead, cadmium, and mercury) |
| Too much protein | Stay close to your recommended amount of protein per day |

## Incomplete versus Complete Protein

Think of sources of protein like food containing puzzle pieces (amino acids). Some sources of protein have only a few pieces of the puzzle (one or more amino acid is missing). When your body has only part of the puzzle, it cannot use the protein to perform important tasks like rebuilding muscle, repairing damaged cells, or making new proteins. However, incomplete proteins are not useless. Incomplete proteins can bind together to make complete proteins. Below is a list of incomplete proteins:

- Some fruits like apples, avocados, and bananas to name a few

- Some vegetables like asparagus, cauliflower, and sweet potatoes to name a few

- Grains

- Nuts

- Legumes (peanuts and beans)

Most vegetarians get their protein from the sources listed in the previous list. When you eat the recommended daily amount of fruits, vegetables, grains, legumes, and nuts, you will consume most or all of the pieces needed to complete your protein puzzle.

*Complete proteins* contain all the puzzle pieces necessary to make new proteins and repair your body. Remember the benefits of protein? Complete sources include:

- Meat
- Fish
- Poultry
- Eggs
- Dairy

Consuming a variety is a sure way to receive other important nutrients like iron and B vitamins in addition to protein. Practice choosing one serving of protein for every meal and snack and you will have a well-balanced, completed puzzle for your body's health.

## Protein and Weight Management

Remember, more calories are required to break down and digest protein than to break down and absorb simple carbohydrates and sugar. Therefore, when you are consuming protein for fuel, you are burning more calories. As we learned in Chapter 1, calories matter. Sources of protein usually have higher calories than sources of carbohydrates (i.e., vegetables), but calories from protein fill you and leave you feeling satisfied longer. As a result, you will not be so preoccupied with your next meal or snack due to overwhelming hunger. Our food should nourish us, fuel us, and satisfy our hunger and our cravings. Diet food that is low in calories and nearly void of nutrients simply gives you something to chew on (or drink in a shake). However, keeping your mouth busy without the necessary nutrition does not mean you are going to maintain or lose weight. Quite the opposite: Chewing on empty calories usually leaves you in a state of depravity.

## Quick and Easy Protein-Packed Dinners

Does ordering a pizza ever seem easier than cooking a healthy, protein-packed meal? Mealtimes are moments of opportunity: You can turn your body into a fat-burning machine with healthy, home-cooked meals *or* you can allow your body to store almost everything you eat as fat with junk food meal choices.

**Tip from Your Trainer:** Use these quick and easy meal ideas to incorporate healthy protein into your day. Substitute any of the

*If there is one thing I have learned from years of battling unstable blood sugar, especially now as an expecting mother, it is that quality protein is essential to my health. Protein keeps me full and satisfied, which helps me embrace life with a clear mind.*

CAITLYN H.
INFIT CLIENT

protein in these recipes with wild-caught fish or grass-fed beef for a delicious variety of protein and heart-healthy omegas.

## 1. Chicken Braised in Liquid Aminos* and Lemon Juice

Serves 4

| | | |
|---|---|---|
| Liquid aminos* | Cayenne pepper flakes | 1 clove garlic |
| Virgin olive oil | Organic sucanat | 1 lemon |

1 pound bone-in chicken (nitrite and nitrate free)

Brown bone-in chicken pieces in a few tablespoons of virgin olive oil. Remove and stir in 1 tablespoon chopped garlic. Add the minced zest of a lemon, a pinch of cayenne, 2 tablespoons liquid aminos, 1 teaspoon organic sucanat**, and 1/3 cup water; stir. Add the chicken, cover, and simmer. Turn the pieces once; the dish will be done in about 15 minutes. Add lemon juice and liquid aminos to taste.

*Liquid aminos are a soy sauce alternative. One brand is Bragg®.

**Organic sucanat is an alternative for table sugar. It is dehydrated cane juice, sweet and packed with nutrients.

## 2. Grilled Chicken with Pesto Sauce

Serves 4

| | | |
|---|---|---|
| 2 cups fresh basil | 1 clove garlic | Sea salt and pepper |
| Pine nuts | Parmesan cheese | Virgin olive oil |

1 pound chicken cutlets (nitrite and nitrate free)

To make the pesto, puree 2 cups fresh basil, 1 garlic clove, a pinch of sea salt, 2 tablespoons pine nuts, 1/2 cup grated Parmesan, and 1/2 cup virgin olive oil in a blender or food processor.

Season 1 pound chicken cutlets with sea salt and pepper. Grill them, turning once, about 8 minutes total. Paint with pesto and serve.

## 3. Stir-Fried Spicy Beef

Serves 4

Liquid aminos are a soy sauce alternative. One brand is Bragg®.

| | | |
|---|---|---|
| 1 pound flank steak | 1/2 cup basil | 1 clove garlic |
| Unrefined coconut oil | Red pepper flakes | Liquid aminos |
| 1 lime or lemon | | |

Thinly slice 1 pound of flank steak across the grain into bite-size pieces. Chop 1/2 cup basil and mix with beef, set aside. Cook 1 1/2 tablespoons minced garlic in 1 tablespoon of coconut oil until slightly brown.

*Most healthy recipes take less time to prepare than waiting for pizza delivery.*

*Did You Know?*

*Protein rebuilds and repairs all cells, not just muscle cells.*

Add beef-basil mixture and 1/4 tablespoon red pepper flakes; cook for 2 minutes. Add 1 tablespoon liquid aminos and the juice of half a lime or lemon and serve.

## 4. Chicken with Citrus Glaze

Serves 4

2 lemons, 1 orange, and 1 grapefruit

Virgin olive oil

1 clove garlic, Fresh thyme leaves, Sea salt and pepper

1 small onion

4 boneless chicken breasts (nitrite and nitrate free)

To make the sauce, warm the zest and juice of one lemon, plus the sections of another lemon, an orange, and a grapefruit in a pan. Add 1/4 cup virgin olive oil, 1 teaspoon fresh thyme leaves, 1/2 teaspoon minced garlic, one small minced onion, sea salt, and pepper. Rub boneless chicken with olive oil and sprinkle with sea salt and pepper. Broil or grill. Serve with the citrus sauce.

## 5. Chicken Tikka with Greek Yogurt Sauce

Serves 4

Low sugar, plain Greek yogurt

Ground cashews

4 boneless chicken breasts (nitrite and nitrate free)

1 clove garlic

Spices: cardamom, coriander, ginger, sea salt and pepper

Cut boneless chicken into 1-inch chunks. Combine with 1/4 cup low-sugar, plain Greek yogurt, 1/4 cup ground cashews, and 1 teaspoon each ground cardamom, ground coriander, minced ginger, and minced garlic. Remove chicken from the marinade and grill until brown and cooked through. To make the sauce, mix 1 cup yogurt with 1 teaspoon minced garlic and some lemon juice, salt, and pepper. Serve with the chicken.

*Most healthy recipes take less time to prepare than waiting for pizza delivery.* As you can see, many of these recipes call for the same or similar ingredients. You could buy two or three pounds of chicken, several citrus fruits, virgin or extra-virgin olive oil, garlic, and a few other spices, and have *several different dinner ideas*, all filled with healthy protein for the week (not to mention leftovers!). Add a side of steamed veggies with different spices to each entrée and you will seldom get bored with your food. Our bodies need protein to perform vital cell repair *and* keep us in check with a healthy weight. If you are not already doing so, add a source of protein to each meal and snack to stay healthy and satisfied throughout the day.

## Practice

*1. Macro nutrient tracking. If you are not already doing this, track your grams of protein per day for three days. Record it here:*

Day 1 _____ grams Are you over/under? _____ grams

Day 2 _____ grams Are you over/under? _____ grams

Day 3 _____ grams Are you over/under? _____ grams

What did you find? Were you surprised?

_____

*2. Be brave! Try a new source of plant or animal protein this week. What did you try?*

_____

*3. Plan ahead. Prepare a recipe with protein and vegetables as the main meal. What did you make?*

_____

*Remember, protein rebuilds and repairs all cells, not just muscle cells.* Getting enough of the right sources of protein is a vital part of your healthy road map to success.

## S2L

Discuss with someone the approximate amount of protein he or she needs per day. Teach them about incomplete versus complete protein sources and share the benefits of protein. Finally, teach him or her the weight management benefits of consuming protein. Determine how many grams he or she needs per day:

_____ grams of protein

# InFIT Workout 4

First time (set) through: Warm up: Go through all of the exercises slowly, 15-20 repetitions each, with no resistance (no weight), 5-10 minutes. Second set: Perform the exercises one at a time, with resistance when appropriate, starting with one lower body exercise, one upper body exercise, and one core exercise with minimal rest in between. Perform all nine exercises and then repeat as your fitness goals and time permit! Tempo: Count to four as you contract (tighten) your muscles during an exercise (exhale); release the exercise on a count of one (inhale). For example, count to four as you lower into a squat and count to one as you stand up. Remember to drink water during your workout and stretch tight muscles.

## Lower Body

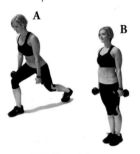

**DB Front Lunge**

|  | Set 1 | Set 2 |
|---|---|---|
| Weight |  |  |
| Reps |  |  |

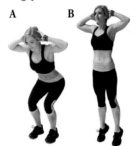

**Prisoner Squat to Toes**

|  | Set 1 | Set 2 |
|---|---|---|
| Weight |  |  |
| Reps |  |  |

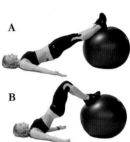

**SB Hamstring Curl**

|  | Set 1 | Set 2 |
|---|---|---|
| Weight |  |  |
| Reps |  |  |

## Upper Body

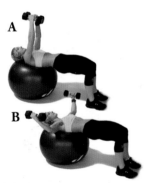

**DB SB Chest Fly**

|  | Set 1 | Set 2 |
|---|---|---|
| Weight |  |  |
| Reps |  |  |

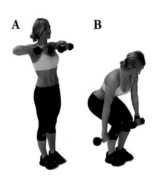

**DB Upright Row**

|  | Set 1 | Set 2 |
|---|---|---|
| Weight |  |  |
| Reps |  |  |

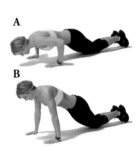

**Knee Triceps Pushup**

|  | Set 1 | Set 2 |
|---|---|---|
| Weight |  |  |
| Reps |  |  |

## Core

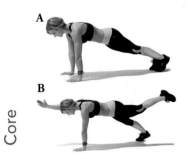

**Prone Arm/Opposite Leg Raise**

|  | Set 1 | Set 2 |
|---|---|---|
| Weight |  |  |
| Reps |  |  |

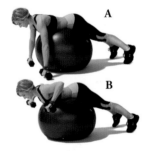

**DB SB Row**

|  | Set 1 | Set 2 |
|---|---|---|
| Weight |  |  |
| Reps |  |  |

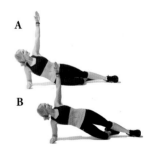

**Knee Side Plank**

|  | Set 1 | Set 2 |
|---|---|---|
| Weight |  |  |
| Reps |  |  |

# InFIT Workout 4—Option II

Have you ever heard of muscle confusion? Your muscles plateau when they are repeatedly exposed to the same movement patterns. Changing the tempo of your exercises is a great way to offer variety in your workouts and break through plateaus in your strength gains and weight loss achievements. Perform all nine exercises and then repeat as your fitness goals and time permit! **Tempo**: Count to four as you contract (tighten) your muscles during an exercise (exhale); release the exercise on a count of one (inhale). For example, count to four as you lower into a squat and count to one as you stand up. Remember to drink water during your workout and stretch tight muscles.

**Lower Body**

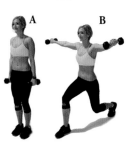

**DB Front Lunge with Lateral Raise**

|  | Set 1 | Set 2 |
|---|---|---|
| Weight |  |  |
| Reps |  |  |

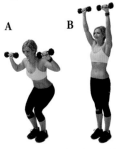

**DB Squat with Shoulder Press**

|  | Set 1 | Set 2 |
|---|---|---|
| Weight |  |  |
| Reps |  |  |

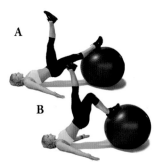

**SB Hamstring Curl—Single Leg**

|  | Set 1 | Set 2 |
|---|---|---|
| Weight |  |  |
| Reps |  |  |

**Upper Body**

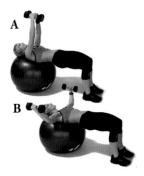

**DB SB Chest Fly—Heavier Weight**

|  | Set 1 | Set 2 |
|---|---|---|
| Weight |  |  |
| Reps |  |  |

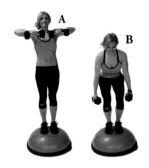

**BOSU DB Upright Row**

|  | Set 1 | Set 2 |
|---|---|---|
| Weight |  |  |
| Reps |  |  |

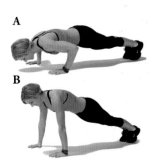

**Full Triceps Pushup**

|  | Set 1 | Set 2 |
|---|---|---|
| Weight |  |  |
| Reps |  |  |

**Core**

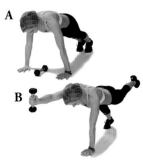

**DB Prone Arm/Opposite Leg Raise**

|  | Set 1 | Set 2 |
|---|---|---|
| Weight |  |  |
| Reps |  |  |

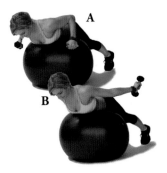

**DB SB Row to Cobra**

|  | Set 1 | Set 2 |
|---|---|---|
| Weight |  |  |
| Reps |  |  |

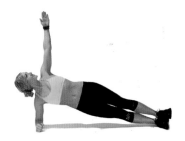

**Full Side Plank**

|  | Set 1 | Set 2 |
|---|---|---|
| Weight |  |  |
| Reps |  |  |

## Review Your Map–Chapter Reflection

Use this road map as a weekly check-in to measure your goals and progress. Fill in the blank spaces at the bottom of the chart to create your own goals. The more often you check in with yourself, the more often you will bring health to the front of your mind, creating intention and success.

| | GOAL | MON | TUE | WED | THU | FRI | SAT | SUN |
| --- | --- | --- | --- | --- | --- | --- | --- | --- |
| | | Actual | Actual | Actual | Actual | Actual | Actual | Actual |
| **Servings of produce (Ch 5)** | | | | | | | | |
| **Water in ounces** | | | | | | | | |
| **Hours of sleep (Ch 2)** | | | | | | | | |
| **Minutes of exercise** | | | | | | | | |
| **Weight** | | | | | | | | |
| **Amount of meals/ snacks per day (Ch 3)** | | | | | | | | |
| **Calories** | | | | | | | | |
| **Number of simple carbs (Ch 6)** | | | | | | | | |
| **Body fat % (optional)** | | | | | | | | |
| **Bowel movements (Ch 8)** | | | | | | | | |
| **Add your own below** | | | | | | | | |
| | | | | | | | | |
| | | | | | | | | |
| | | | | | | | | |

Did you achieve most of your goals? _____ Why? _____

What is your plan for the next week to either stay on your original course or modify based on this week's review?

How do you feel about your progress thus far?

# LIVING AFFIRMATION
## WELLNESS FOR YOUR SOUL

## Surrender When You Do Not Understand

Jesus: "I am the living bread which came down from heaven. If anyone eats of this bread, he will live forever; and the bread that I shall give is My flesh, which I shall give for the life of the world." The Jews therefore quarreled among themselves, saying, "How can this Man give us *His* flesh to eat?" John 6:51-52

Understandably, the Jews were confused by Jesus' words in the scripture verse. But how did they respond? Instead of voicing their confusion and frustration to God, they quarreled amongst themselves and left. We still behave like this today when we get upset.

*What confuses and frustrates you about God?*

I am talking about a situation that keeps you from fully surrendering your trust and hope to God: a job loss? A death? A serious illness? A rebellious child?

We have two choices: 1. Respond with denial and/or anger. 2. Talk to God. Tell God you are confused and frustrated. Allow God to respond to you and be surprised when you pay attention.

*Do you have a situation in your life that you need to bring to God?* Surrendering means that you can experience deeper intimacy, peace, and freedom with God, who already knows what frustrates us. Vulnerability and humility changes our hearts when we go to God. He desires to heal us from the pain that comes from our lack of understanding.

My prayer for you is to surrender your frustrations to God and experience the healing touch in parts of your life that you do not fully understand, instead of walking out on the relationship.

Be blessed abundantly! ~ *Christina Zaczkowski*, MA, CPT

## *Reflection*

_____

_____

_____

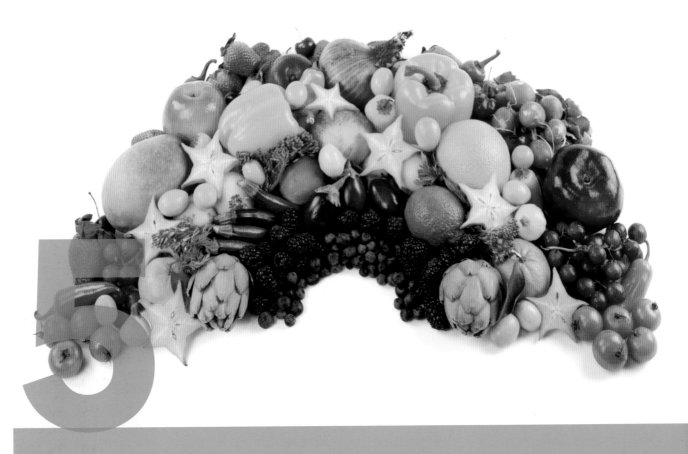

# EAT A RAINBOW FOR WEIGHT LOSS

## Principle Questions:

1. Why are fruits and vegetables essential to your health and weight?

2. How many servings do you need and what is considered a serving size?

3. Why is eating a variety of produce important?

4. What are the best sources of produce?

5. Is it more expensive to eat clean?

Eat a rainbow. The first time I was introduced to that phrase, it stuck. Did you know that the rainbow is a sign of God's covenant with Noah after the flood? In the same sense, make a covenant with your health by cherishing the rainbow of fruits and vegetables!

I encourage you to eat a rainbow as often as possible (at least every two days would be ideal). To make it even simpler, eat at least *one fruit and/or vegetable with every meal and snack*. Let's break that down.

Why did I specifically say to eat a rainbow? Why not eat fruits with the most antioxidants and vegetables that are highest in fiber? Or buy produce that is on sale? Those are all great places to start, *but the key to produce is in the nutrients*. When you eat a variety of colorful produce, you are ensuring a wide range of vitamins and minerals that your body *needs and longs for*. If you eat broccoli and spinach and green peppers all day, you will be well sourced in vitamin C and vitamin K, but you would be lacking vitamins A and E, which are found in orange vegetables and fruit like carrots and dried apricots. When you eat a rainbow every couple of days, you consume nourishment to fuel every cell in your body. Vitamins, minerals, and macro nutrients make up the individual composition of our DNA. When we lack essential nutrients, illness, disease, and pain find opportunities to creep in and attack our bodies.

## Benefits of Produce

In Chapter 2 we looked at eating for fuel *and* nourishment. Produce gives us clean fuel and ample nourishment. The benefits of eating a variety of fruits and vegetables include:

- Reduced risk of disease, diabetes, and high blood pressure. Fruits and vegetables (organic when available) help to keep you out of the doctor's office.

- Vitamins and minerals—healthy and energizing, a perfect combination

- Convenience—after you wash them, you can just grab and go! Apples in the purse, a bag of carrots in the diaper bag, or an orange in the brief case. Produce travels well.

- Low calories—most produce is low in calories and high in satisfaction

- Antioxidants—help to remove disease-causing free radicals from your body

**Weight Management Benefit:**

Produce fills you up and is low in calories.

Tip from Your Trainer: Eat seasonal produce. It usually contains nutrients you need seasonally. Example: The vitamin D in squash helps your body store the vitamin through the winter, especially if you live in a cold climate where you may not get regular sun exposure.

Tip from Your Trainer: Notice how you can eat certain packaged foods like ice cream and chips until the package is empty? When was the last time you finished the entire bag of lettuce or polished off three apples? If you still crave certain foods after one serving, it may be time to pick a different food. Produce is satisfying.

- Tons of fiber—natural fiber your body can break down and digest without creating a laxative effect

- Water—most are high in water content, making fruits and vegetables their own perfect delivery system to get water-soluble nutrients to the cells

- Added color and texture to your meals—presentation goes a long way. Make your meals visibly appealing and you (and your family) will be more likely to enjoy them.

## Weight Management

Look how much more enticing is the grilled basket of vegetables over the greasy cheeseburger on a white bun.

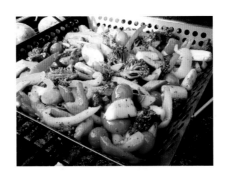

*The Grill Basket: Approximately 300 Calories*

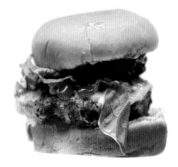

*One Cheeseburger: 1,200+ Calories*

Fruits and vegetables, especially vegetables, are one of the most important components to losing weight and maintaining your ideal weight. Again, look at the pictures of the grill basket of veggies versus the dripping greasy burger. You can see the difference in nourishment. By eating a healthy volume of vegetables, you will nourish your body with essential vitamins and minerals, fuel up with fiber for healthy digestion, and protect your cells from the leading causes of death and diseases—with minimum calories. *If we did nothing else but move our bodies more often, remove added sugar from our diets, and ate a variety of vegetables every day, 80% of the leading causes of death and disease would disappear.* This proven, successful secret requires lifestyle changes, but the results ensure a healthy weight, abundant energy, and less disease. Produce is one food group where I do not negotiate. If you do not like the taste of fruits and vegetables, eat them

### Should You Go Organic?

When choosing produce, always look for certified organic products. Most non-organic produce carries potential chemicals like pesticides, herbicides, and preservatives that are harmful to your thyroid and metabolism. These chemicals are also linked to chronic inflammation, which is a contributing factor to most leading causes of death and disease. If 100% organic produce is not in the budget, choose organic when the skin of the fruit or vegetable is consumed, such as apples and celery.

*"But until a person can say deeply and honestly, 'I am what I am today because of the choices I made yesterday,' that person cannot say, "I choose otherwise."*

STEPHEN R. COVEY

milk for regular milk. However, unsweetened almond milk offers calcium without added chemicals often found in cow milk, and avoiding dairy may be more beneficial for individuals with asthma and certain respiratory and skin conditions.

Canned fruit is a good source when you are out of fresh or frozen fruit. Canned fruit is also nice to have on hand if you cannot get to the grocery store, if your budget does not allow you to always buy fresh, or if you do not have time to go buy fresh fruit. Also, choose fruit that is canned with 100% fruit juice rather than heavy syrup or lite syrup. The price is usually the same, but the health benefits of fruit are lessened when drenched in sticky, sugary corn syrup. Canned fruit is great on its own or paired with cottage cheese, yogurt, or salad. Children and mature adults sometimes prefer canned fruit because it is much softer and easier to eat. However, choose canned produce sparingly to avoid excess aluminum ingestion. Aluminum is a heavy metal that is great for canning, but not great for our bodies. Do not rely on canned goods as your main source of produce.

Dried or dehydrated fruits are great for salads, yogurt embellishments, homemade trail mixes, rice pilafs, and homemade baked goods (among others). Dried cranberries and cherries are great for all the above ideas. Dried blueberries are great in granola or baked goods. Dried bananas and plantains are good for salty snacking, and dried tropical fruit makes for great dessert alone or with yogurt. Dried fruits often contain large amounts of added sugar, so use them in moderation.

## Veggies, Veggies, and More Veggies

I have also detailed a list of vegetables that are available at most grocery stores so that you can add something new to your veggie repertoire. Make it a goal to eat at least one veggie daily at every meal and snack!

- Artichoke, arugula, asparagus, bamboo, beans, beet, bok choy, broccoli, Brussels sprouts, cabbage, capers, carrot, celery, chard, collards, corn, cucumber, eggplant, endive, fennel, garbanzo, garlic, ginger, ginseng, horseradish, jicama, jojoba, kale, leek, lentils, lettuce, melon, mushroom, okra, onion, paprika, parsley, parsnip, peas, pepper, pimiento, potato, pumpkin, radicchio, radish, rhubarb, romaine lettuce, rutabaga, saffron, sea kale, shallot, soybeans, spinach, squash, sweet potato, and yams

What are different forms of vegetables?

What are your favorite vegetables?

What new vegetable will you try this week?

*The practical information from* Living Wellness *flows right into my cooking! Exploring "eating a rainbow" has been so much fun for my entire family. We are drawn to the table by the colorful sight before us and then the discovery of what each color tastes like begins. Cooking to appeal every sense makes eating for fuel and nourishment even more enjoyable for us all.*

TRACY R.
INFIT DIRECTOR

A. Fresh        B. Frozen

C. Canned       D. Dried

Fresh is usually best, but variety is always wise! Stock up on fresh, frozen, canned, and dried to provide texture and taste into every meal and snack.

What can you do with your favorite vegetables?

## Salad Recipe

Original recipe modified from Williams-Sonoma *Salad of the Day*

## Roasted Sweet Potato Salad with Pecans and Green Onions

*This colorful roasted root, vegetable salad is delicious alongside broiled steaks or oven-baked ribs. Use any variety of sweet potato you like, including the ones sometimes labeled "garnet yams," which have a bright orange color and moist, sweet flesh.*

Serves 4-6

3 pounds (1.5 kilograms) sweet potatoes

2 tablespoons virgin olive oil

Mineral salt and pre-ground pepper

1/2 cup pecans

1/3 cup fresh lime juice

3 tablespoons real maple syrup

1/2 cup minced green onions, including tender green parts

3-4 leaves kale, stemmed and leaves torn

Preheat the oven to 400 degrees Fahrenheit. Peel the sweet potatoes and cut them into 1-inch chunks. Put them in a large baking pan, drizzle with 1 1/2 tablespoons of the oil, sprinkle with 1/2 teaspoon salt, and mix to coat. Spread the sweet potatoes in a single layer and roast, stirring occasionally until tender when pierced with a knife, 25-30 minutes.

Meanwhile, in a dry frying pan, toast the pecans over medium-low heat, stirring, until fragrant and starting to brown, about 5 minutes. Pour onto a plate to cool.

In a large bowl, mix the lime juice, maple syrup, and remaining 1/2 tablespoon oil. Add the hot roasted sweet potatoes to the lime juice mixture along with the pecans, green onions, and torn kale. Mix well and season with pepper and additional salt. Serve at once or let cool to room temperature and mix again before serving.

## Stir Fry Recipe

Original recipe modified from Williams-Sonoma

Serves 4

2 tablespoons virgin or extra coconut oil

1 red bell pepper, cored, seeded, and julienned

1 yellow bell pepper, cored, seeded, and julienned

1/2 cup red onion, thinly sliced

1 cup yellow squash, half-moon sliced

1 cup small broccoli florets

1 baby eggplant, cut into chunks

8 ounces chicken or steak, cut into large chunks

1 clove garlic, minced

1/2 cup teriyaki sauce (check the label: no more than 2 grams sugar per serving)

2 cups sliced bok choy

1 cup fresh mung bean sprouts

1/4 teaspoon freshly ground black pepper

1/4 teaspoon mineral salt

1/2 cup snow peas

2 tablespoons sesame oil

Start by preparing and cutting all the vegetables and measuring your ingredients so that they are ready to go. Once you begin stir-frying, the next steps go quickly.

In a wok or large skillet, heat coconut oil over high heat until almost smoking. Add the peppers and onion while stirring constantly. Add successively the squash, broccoli, eggplant, chicken or steak, garlic, and teriyaki sauce. Cook, stirring constantly for 2 minutes. Add the bok choy, sprouts, pepper, and salt and cook, stirring, until crisp-tender, about 2 minutes more.

Stir in snow peas and sesame oil and remove from heat. Serve immediately.

## Grilled Fish and Summer Squash

Serves 4

2 teaspoons Dijon mustard

Lemon zest, grated from 1 lemon

2 tablespoons fresh lemon juice

1/3 cup (plus more as needed) virgin or extra virgin olive oil

1 small Serrano chili, seeded and minced

1 teaspoon minced fresh marjoram

1 teaspoon minced fresh basil

Coarse mineral salt and fresh ground pepper

1 pound of your favorite fish, cut in chunks (mahi mahi works well for skewers)

8 summer squash, cut lengthwise into 3 pieces each

Soak bamboo skewers in water and cover for 30 minutes. Prepare a charcoal or gas grill for direct-heat cooking over medium-high heat.

Add the mustard to a small bowl and stir in lemon zest and juice, mixing well. Gradually whisk in 1/3 cup olive oil. Mix in the chili and herbs. Season the sauce to taste with salt and pepper.

Arrange the squash on the grill, cover, and cook until tender and lightly charred, about 5 minutes per side. Transfer to a plate. Place the fish on the grill, on the skewers, and cook, uncovered, until just cooked through, about 4 minutes per side. Remove the fish from the skewers and cut the squash crosswise. Transfer the fish and squash to

Let's add up all the money we just saved by consistently eating clean.

- How much would you save per week if you cut down on junk food, fast food, and eating out?

- How much would you save if you did not miss work due to your (or your child's) illness?

- How much would you save if you did not buy fiber supplements, weight loss pills, or diet programs?

- How much would you save if you did not need a sleep study or drugs to help you sleep (or help you snore less)?

- How much would you save if you did not need drugs to keep you awake? Gourmet coffee is expensive.

- How much would you save if you did not need mood-altering drugs?

- How much would you save if you did not have to buy larger clothes?

- How much would you save if you did not have to go to the doctor as often?

a medium bowl and toss with the lemon-herb sauce. Season to taste with salt and pepper and serve right away.

**Quick Tips: Vary the recipe by using red bell peppers in place of summer squash or scallops instead of fish.** Chicken breasts are also good with these seasonings. To save time, make the dressing one day ahead and refrigerate. Bring it to room temperature before using.

Canned vegetables can be good to throw into a stir fry when you are low on fresh veggies and are also great on a salad; try canned artichoke hearts on your favorite salad for a boost of protein (yes, protein!), vitamin C, vitamin K, folate (good for the brain), magnesium, omegas, and fiber–wow! All this from a canned veggie (or fresh if you prepare artichoke hearts)! These nutrients fuel your body, protect your brain, and keep your body free from disease and malnourishment.

Dried veggies are also great for snacking. Dehydrated green beans and snap peas are popular among my colleagues for their flavor, texture, and healthy qualities. Dried beans are a wonderful addition to soups, salads, wraps, and a stir fry (you will need to first soak and cook dried beans).

How many vegetable servings do you need per day?

**Trainer's Recommendation:** You need at least three to five servings of veggies per day (seven to nine servings of produce total).

## Eating Clean–Is It More Expensive?

Most fruits and veggies are low in calories and high in nourishment (Chapter 2). Produce also supplies heart-healthy fiber, which is responsible for absorbing toxins and sweeping them out of our body.

I often hear that eating healthy is too expensive. This is simply not true. Initially, we may take more time to learn how to grocery shop and cook with healthy ingredients, but eating clean, whole foods is *not* more expensive. How much money do we spend on empty calorie foods: chips, ice cream, soda, candy bars in the checkout lane? One bag of chips can cost more than three dollars . . . for just 7 ounces, versus similar spending on a half dozen organic peaches in season. Replacing junk food with whole food provides cost savings *now* and long-term: Consuming healthy food allows us to be more productive at home and work, sleep better, have less mental health problems, and manage our ideal weight.

In my experience, better health reduces medical bills. Think of consuming quality produce as an investment into your health.

**The cost savings from eating clean are tangible**. *They are not just produce-in-the-sky suggestions that may or may not happen with improved health. When you fuel and nourish your body with the right foods and the right amounts, you* will *be healthier. You* will *feel better. You* will *save money, short-term and long-term.*

## Practice

Make sure that *every* meal and snack includes either a fruit and/or a vegetable every day.

1. Count your daily intake of produce for three days and record it here:

Day 1

Day 2

Day 3

2. Try a new fruit and veggie this week. What did you try?

New fruit:

New vegetable:

Example produce plan:

- Orange with breakfast

- Apple with mid-morning snack

- Spinach with lunch

- Broccoli and carrots with mid-day snack

- Sliced red peppers and snap peas with dinner

The plan above offers a minimum of five to seven servings of fruits and veggies *per day*. If one of your goals is weight management, this plan *likely* replaces other high-calorie, low-nutrition choices. Additionally, the plan of one fruit and/or veggie with every meal and snack adds abundant nourishment. Get in the habit of eating a rainbow often and you will certainly glow with radiant health. When your produce consumption is balanced, weight management is naturally easier.

**S2L**

What did you learn in this chapter about fruits and vegetables?

Were you surprised when you counted how many servings you consumed per day of each? Yes/No

Teach someone how many servings of fruits and vegetables they need per day and how simple it can be to get them.

Who will you teach?

Share recipes and meal plans with friends that use vegetables as the main course.

# InFIT Workout 5

First time (set) through: Warm up: Go through all of the exercises slowly, 15-20 repetitions each, with no resistance (no weight), 5-10 minutes. Second set: In the Strength Level, we transition from performing one exercise in each row to performing all three exercises in each row before moving on to the next muscle group (Lower Body, Upper Body, and Core) with minimal rest in between exercises. Perform all nine exercises and then repeat as your fitness goals and time permit! *The goal in the Strength Level is to fatigue (exhaust the muscle) after no more than 12 reps. If you can do more than 12 reps per exercise, increase your weight or move to the exercises in Option II.* If a particular exercise or workout causes pain to your joints, *skip it* and move to the next (or previous) exercise or workout. If this phase is too difficult, return to the previous phase until you feel more comfortable advancing. These workouts are designed to develop stronger, more flexible, and more toned muscles.

## Lower Body

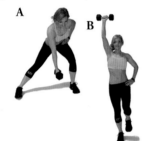

**DB Lateral Lunge to Single Arm Press**

|  | Set 1 | Set 2 |
|---|---|---|
| Weight |  |  |
| Reps |  |  |

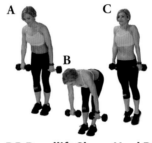

**DB Deadlift Shrug Heel Raise**

|  | Set 1 | Set 2 |
|---|---|---|
| Weight |  |  |
| Reps |  |  |

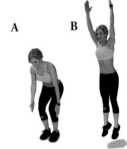

**Squat Jump**

|  | Set 1 | Set 2 |
|---|---|---|
| Weight |  |  |
| Reps |  |  |

## Upper Body

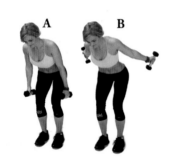

**DB ISO Squat with Cobra**

|  | Set 1 | Set 2 |
|---|---|---|
| Weight |  |  |
| Reps |  |  |

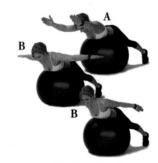

**SB Combo 1**

|  | Set 1 | Set 2 |
|---|---|---|
| Weight |  |  |
| Reps |  |  |

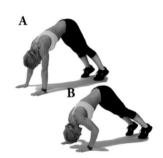

**Inverted Pushup**

|  | Set 1 | Set 2 |
|---|---|---|
| Weight |  |  |
| Reps |  |  |

## Core

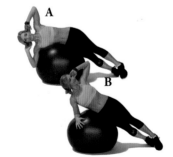

**SB Side Crunch**

|  | Set 1 | Set 2 |
|---|---|---|
| Weight |  |  |
| Reps |  |  |

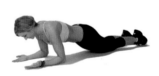

**Knee Plank**

|  | Set 1 | Set 2 |
|---|---|---|
| Weight |  |  |
| Reps |  |  |

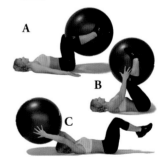

**SB Pass**

|  | Set 1 | Set 2 |
|---|---|---|
| Weight |  |  |
| Reps |  |  |

# InFIT Workout 5—Option II

During the strength level (next for workouts), we continue building strength on the strong foundation you have developed, and increase your core muscles, balance, and strength. *The goal in the Strength Level is to fatigue (exhaust the muscle) after no more than 12 reps. If you can do more than 12 reps per exercise, increase your weight.* In the Strength Level, we transition from performing one exercise in each row to performing all three exercises in each row before moving on to the next muscle group (Lower Body, Upper Body, and Core) with minimal rest in between exercises.

Lower Body

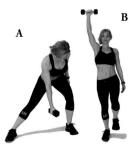

**DB Lateral Lunge to Single Arm Press**

|         | Set 1 | Set 2 |
|---------|-------|-------|
| Weight  |       |       |
| Reps    |       |       |

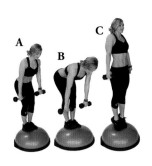

**BOSU DB Deadlift Shrug to Toes**

|         | Set 1 | Set 2 |
|---------|-------|-------|
| Weight  |       |       |
| Reps    |       |       |

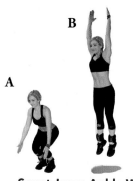

**Squat Jump Ankle Weights**

|         | Set 1 | Set 2 |
|---------|-------|-------|
| Weight  |       |       |
| Reps    |       |       |

Upper Body

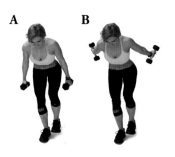

**DB ISO Squat with Cobra—Single Leg**

|         | Set 1 | Set 2 |
|---------|-------|-------|
| Weight  |       |       |
| Reps    |       |       |

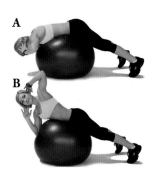

**SB Back Extension with Rotation**

|         | Set 1 | Set 2 |
|---------|-------|-------|
| Weight  |       |       |
| Reps    |       |       |

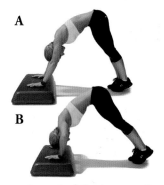

**Inverted Pushup on Step**

|         | Set 1 | Set 2 |
|---------|-------|-------|
| Weight  |       |       |
| Reps    |       |       |

Core

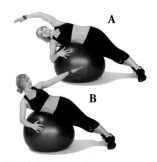

**SB Side Crunch Long Lever**

|         | Set 1 | Set 2 |
|---------|-------|-------|
| Weight  |       |       |
| Reps    |       |       |

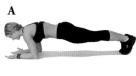
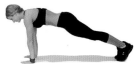

**Full Body Plank**

|         | Set 1 | Set 2 |
|---------|-------|-------|
| Weight  |       |       |
| Reps    |       |       |

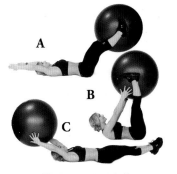

**SB Pass—Straight Leg**

|         | Set 1 | Set 2 |
|---------|-------|-------|
| Weight  |       |       |
| Reps    |       |       |

## Review Your Map—Chapter Reflection

Use this road map as a weekly check-in to measure your goals and progress. Fill in the blank spaces at the bottom of the chart to create your own goals. The more often you check in with yourself, the more often you will bring health to the front of your mind, creating intention and success.

| | GOAL | MON Actual | TUE Actual | WED Actual | THU Actual | FRI Actual | SAT Actual | SUN Actual |
|---|---|---|---|---|---|---|---|---|
| Servings of produce (Ch 5) | | | | | | | | |
| Water in ounces | | | | | | | | |
| Hours of sleep (Ch 2) | | | | | | | | |
| Minutes of exercise | | | | | | | | |
| Weight | | | | | | | | |
| Amount of meals/ snacks per day (Ch 3) | | | | | | | | |
| Calories | | | | | | | | |
| Number of simple carbs (Ch 6) | | | | | | | | |
| Body fat % (optional) | | | | | | | | |
| Bowel movements (Ch 8) | | | | | | | | |
| **Add your own below** | | | | | | | | |
| | | | | | | | | |
| | | | | | | | | |
| | | | | | | | | |

Did you achieve most of your goals? _____ Why? _____

What is your plan for the next week to either stay on your original course or modify based on this week's review?

How do you feel about your progress thus far?

# LIVING AFFIRMATION
### WELLNESS FOR YOUR SOUL

## Organically Grown

To everything there is a season, a time for every purpose under heaven. Ecclesiastes 3:1

Chapter 5 encourages us to consume organic produce. Why? Because life is more comparable to a tomato than a box of chocolates.

A conventionally grown tomato grows in overexploited, nutrient-scarce soil to meet the demands of consumers. Nutrient-scarce soil grows a nutrient-scarce tomato. Organically grown tomatoes are grown in nutrient-rich soil, making organics some of the healthiest foods on earth.

What is your soil? Does your soil encourage spiritual growth? Do you make room in your busy life for quiet time, meditation, and reflection (nourishment to the soil) or do you continually allow your soil to be overwhelmed with responsibilities, expectations, and overexploited with noise?

A conventionally grown tomato gets plucked and shipped before it is naturally ripened to avoid getting moldy at the grocery store. The tomato is sprayed with argon gas to give the appearance that it ripened on the vine. As the tomato forced to ripen before its time, we have been forced to pretend that everything about our lives is great when sometimes life is not. Media and pop culture tells us that we need to have it all together so we pretend; as the conventionally grown tomato, we airbrush our lives in order to appear perfect. Organic tomatoes are allowed to grow naturally without harmful chemicals. This means they may have an occasional bruise.

But guess what? When it comes to buying tomatoes, I spend more and go organic!

Just as we have the choice to buy produce the way it was intended, organic, we have the ability to grow ourselves organically, meaning there is no artificial expectation on how we turn out. Growing in God offers freedom. No one should be treated as a conventionally grown tomato—not even a tomato!

*Do you feel as though you are out of sync with yourself because of your spray-painted life?* I encourage you to prayerfully meditate and write about your thoughts and feelings on growing fully in your spiritual soil.

Be blessed abundantly! ~ *Christina Zaczkowski*, MA, CPT

## *Reflection*

_____

_____

_____

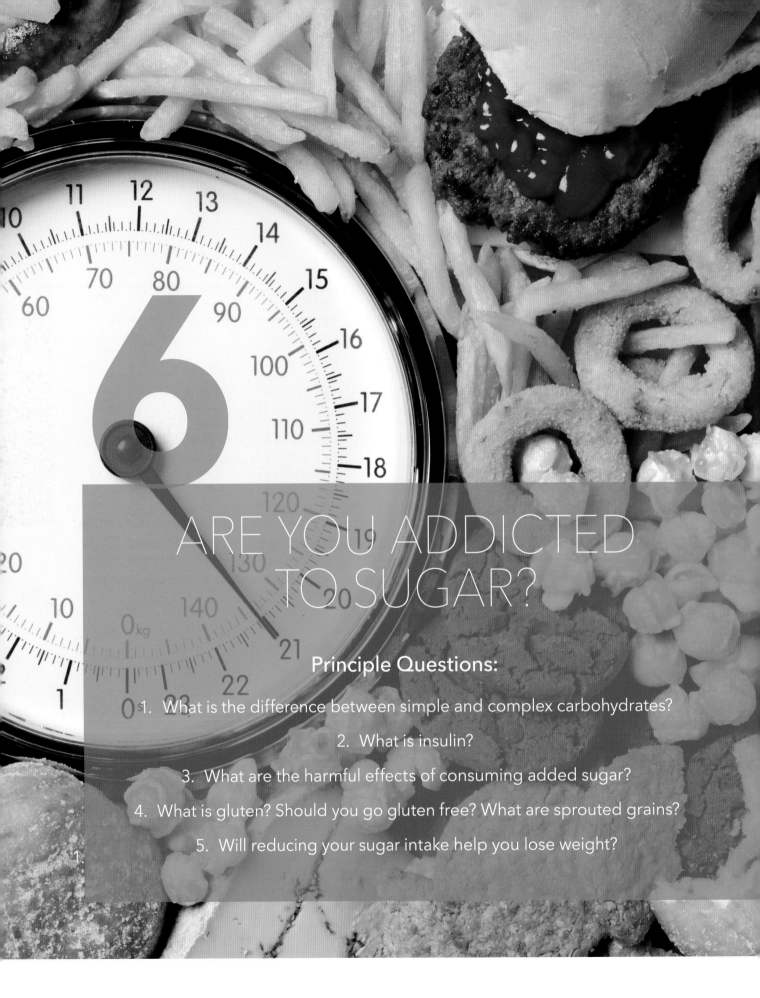

# 6

# ARE YOU ADDICTED TO SUGAR?

**Principle Questions:**

1. What is the difference between simple and complex carbohydrates?

2. What is insulin?

3. What are the harmful effects of consuming added sugar?

4. What is gluten? Should you go gluten free? What are sprouted grains?

5. Will reducing your sugar intake help you lose weight?

We are an over-carbed (over-sugared) nation. We are addicted to sugar. Sugar is killing us, slowly and painfully. There is added sugar in almost every sports drink and alcoholic drink, and now there is even talk of adding sugar to milk! For most individuals, consuming sugar from natural sources has little to no negative effects on the body; it is the overwhelming amount of *added sugar* we consume that is killing us. What does sugar have to do with carbohydrates? Everything.

## Simple versus Complex Carbohydrates

Here is the definition of *simple carbohydrates,* according to Mosby's Dictionary of Complementary and Alternative Medicine, 2005, Elsevier:

*"n.pl sugars—including dextrose, fructose, lactose, maltose, sucrose, white sugar, corn syrup, honey, and turbinado sugar—that are quickly and easily absorbed into the bloodstream."*

Use the definition above when going grocery shopping. Look for added sugars in packaged foods and then *avoid them like a root canal.* Simple carbohydrates (carbs) have the same effect as added sugars in your body. Simple carbs are substances that *turn into sugar* quickly in your body:

- Bread
- Cookies
- Muffins
- Pasta

### The American Heritage definition of *complex carbohydrates* follows:

*Any of a group of organic compounds that includes sugars, starches, cellulose, and gums and serves as a major energy source in the diet of animals. These compounds are produced by photosynthetic plants and contain only carbon, hydrogen, and oxygen, usually in the ratio 1:2:1.*

Complex carbohydrates (carbs) are substances that are *slow* to digest and absorb, allowing your blood sugar to remain balanced and stable. A few examples of complex carbs include:

- Vegetables, sweet potatoes, and white potatoes
- Whole grains
- Legumes

**Additional List of Simple Carbs to Avoid:**

- Table sugar
- Corn syrup (dextrose)
- High fructose corn syrup
- Fruit juice
- Candy
- Cake
- Crackers
- Bread made with white flour
- Pasta made with white flour
- Bagels made with white flour
- Soda and sugary sports drinks
- Candy
- All baked goods made with white flour
- Most packaged cereals
- Processed jam
- Chocolate
- Biscuits

**Complex Carbs (Partial List):**

- Spinach
- Whole barley
- Grapefruit
- Turnip greens
- Buckwheat
- Apples
- Lettuce
- Buckwheat bread
- Prunes
- Watercress
- Dried apricots
- Zucchini
- Oatmeal
- Pears
- Asparagus
- Oat bran cereal
- Plums
- Artichokes
- Muesli
- Strawberries
- Wild rice
- Oranges
- Cabbage
- Brown rice
- Yams
- Celery
- Whole-grain bread
- Cucumbers
- Beans
- Potatoes
- Lentils
- Cauliflower
- Kidney beans
- Eggplant
- Soy milk
- Lentils
- Onions
- Whole meal bread
- Split peas

# What Is the Difference?

Most simple carbs are grains and sugars that *lack* essential nutrients and fiber. Whereas, complex carbs *contain* most of their original, essential nutrients, and fiber. These original nutrients in complex carbs aid in digestion, absorption, and elimination, *rather* than making those processes worse.

The following chart simplifies what happens to our blood sugar when we consume added sugar.

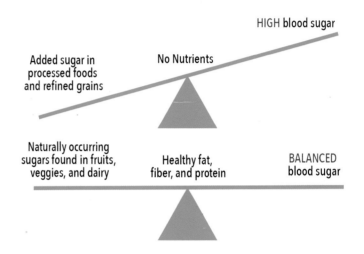

Balanced insulin response
without spiking your blood sugar and allowing
your body ability to use fat as fuel

## Let us look more closely at simple and complex carbohydrates.

Simple carbs turn to sugar in our bodies. Imagine eating a fast-food hamburger and instead of the bun, you ate bun-shaped sugar cubes! Or, instead of a warm bagel with cream cheese you ate a bagel-shaped sugar cube with cream cheese. Or perhaps, the worst is imagining your plate full of pasta noodles turning into—you guessed it, a plate full of sugar cubes drizzled with tomato paste. UGH! When we eat refined or enriched grains, we might as well be eating sugar cubes, void of most digestible and absorbable nutrition.

The challenge of refined grains and simple carbs: Most food with added sugar or foods that turn into sugar quickly in our bodies are high in calories, low in protein, low in fiber, and *not* satisfying (low satiety). We often crave sugar because of the quick energy we feel, but that rush does not last long.

*Overconsuming refined sugar results in a roller coaster of a day — a roller coaster of blood sugar, energy levels, depression, anxiety, hormones, body aches, brain fog, obesity, and disease.* Fat-free cereal or bagel for breakfast, spike and crash; packaged snack cake or candy for a treat, spike and crash; white flour sandwich and soda for lunch, spike and crash. Continuing this pattern results in feeling so hungry by the end of the day that you eat every available packaged food in the pantry. If you took the time to add up all the empty calories from the day, you would most likely be appalled.

Too many high calorie, low satiety foods means weight gain. Repeat.

High-calories, low-satiety means weight gain—We want *more* because the foods and beverages we are consuming lack essential nutrients and keep our bodies in want! Guess what, if you eat like that on a regular basis, you are teaching your body to want junk food, void of anything truly satisfying.

Another factor to consider when consuming simple sugar or carbs is our body's insulin response. When we eat or drink sugar, our body releases insulin to help balance our blood sugar. When we overconsume sugar, the pancreas (organ that produces insulin) has two responses:

1. Gets tired and begins to wear out (non-technical terms) or becomes insulin resistant. This is also known as pre-diabetes. At this point, the damaging effects of diabetes can usually be reversed with proper nutrition. If an individual does not significantly reduce his or her sugar intake (or foods that turn into sugar), diabetes is almost unavoidable.

2. When the pancreas is worn out; then comes Type 2 Diabetes, or insulin dependency. Paying for and becoming dependent on avoidable medication for the rest of your life is expensive and cumbersome.

Our bodies were designed for balanced nutrition. Long-term abuse of *any substance* will have a negative effect on our bodies. Sugar, the sparkling white poison, is one of the worst food substances to abuse.

### Will Your Palate Ever Change?

Yes, yes, and yes! I have seen it again and again. Give it a try! You do not have to give up all simple sugar (although that would not be a terrible idea). Make small changes. Start with reducing added sugar in your breakfast for a few days and work your way up to dinner's dessert.

### Look at Your Plate

List any simple carbs you had yesterday:

Breakfast

Lunch

Dinner

Snacks

## What Are the Harmful Effects of the Sparkling White Poison?

- Chronic diseases
- Diabetes
- High blood pressure
- Chronic inflammation
- Disease
- Increased triglycerides
- Obesity
- Tooth decay

Do you consider yourself having a sweet tooth? Yes/No

How many servings of sugar, grains, bread, et cetera did you have yesterday?

What are a few complex carb alternatives?

## Should You Avoid the Sparkling White Poison?

Yes.

When I encourage clients to avoid sugar or foods that turn to sugar, the panicked question inevitably arises, *What am I going to eat? What am I going to do without my sugary cereal in the morning, white bread at lunch, or sweet treats at Thanksgiving?* My job becomes fun and challenging at this point. Refer back to Chapter 4; I listed dozens of protein sources and five delicious protein-packed recipes. Refer back to Chapter 5. I listed ninety-eight fruits and vegetables available at most grocery stores! There are *so many* healthy foods you can eat without consuming excessive added sugar and simple carbohydrates. As you may have discovered, changing your eating habits takes time, and it will certainly be challenging, but trust me when I say change is possible. *You can do it! You are worth the challenge!* Your health and wellness is worth the struggle! Your pallet will change. Eventually (if you are not already there), you will like and, dare I say, *crave* clean, whole foods over junk food!

## Complex Carbs

Carbs come in two main sources: simple and complex. Complex-carbs are a heart-healthy and weight balancing replacement for added sugar and most simple carbohydrates. The insulin response I refer to above happens when we consume foods that are high in sugar and low or void of natural nutrients and fiber (foods that increase your blood sugar). Complex carbohydrates are balanced, nutritious sources that help to regulate our blood sugar and load us up with vital nutrients. Examples of complex carbohydrates include:

- Vegetables
- Nuts and seeds
- Legumes
- Potatoes
- Milk and dairy
- Whole grains
- Sweet potatoes

**Notes**

*"We were made to crave—long for, want greatly, desire eagerly, and beg for—God. Only God."*

Lysa TerKeurst

# Gluten-Free Grains?

Grains contain a protein called gluten. Do you need to go gluten free? How do you know? What is gluten?

Gluten is a protein found in the grains of wheat, barley, and rye. Think of gluten like glue that holds grains together and gives it a nice texture and smooth flavor. There is nothing inherently harmful with gluten. However, some of our bodies are rejecting gluten as a result of:

- Grossly overeating grains with little to no nutrients

- Eating grains that are genetically modified

- Not eating enough fiber to cleanse our insides

## The two types of people who should **not** eat gluten include:

Individuals who have a sensitivity to and become ill after eating gluten. (Example: After eating grains, there is an onset of an upset stomach, gas, and bloating.) Some experience a flare up in skin conditions like rosacea and dermatitis. Fortunately, these annoying side effects of eating grains do not usually cause permanent damage.

Individuals who have a severe condition called celiac disease. This disease results in damage to the intestines, gastrointestinal distress, and nutritional deficiencies. If left untreated, these reactions can lead to intestinal cancers, osteoporosis, and infertility. An *Archives of Internal Medicine* study in 2003 suggests that celiac disease is far more prevalent than anyone has suspected, affecting 1 in 133 Americans.

If you get ill after eating grains or you suspect you may have celiac disease, consult with your physician.

Some people still get an upset stomach after eating grains even if they are not gluten intolerant or suffering from celiac disease. This uncomfortable condition could be due to your body not breaking down the grain or absorbing all the nutrients properly. If I am describing you, try eating sprouted grains.

# Sprouted Grains, Seeds, and Legumes

We have been sprouting foods for a *long* time, but the evidence coming out in favor of sprouting is growing all the time. Sprouting grains increases the absorption of many of the essential nutrients, including B vitamins, vitamin C, folate, fiber, and essential amino acids, such as lysine, which is often lacking in grains. Many individuals who are not gluten intolerant but still get ill after eating grains switch to sprouted or soaked grains and are pleasantly surprised to feel great, stay satisfied longer, and have better digestion! Because there are no negative side effects of consuming sprouted foods, I recommend replacing your white flour and whole grains with sprouted grain products whenever possible. Food for Life and TruRoots are among a few brands that offer a wonderful variety of sprouted products.

> *"It's not the 'how to' I'm missing. It's the 'want to'. . . really wanting to make changes and deciding that the results of those changes are worth the sacrifice."*
>
> LYSA TERKEURST,
> *MADE TO CRAVE*

Here are just a few more proven reasons to switch to sprouted today:

- Sprouted brown rice reduces the risk of cardiovascular disease.

- Sprouted brown rice fights against diabetes.

- Sprouted buckwheat protects against fatty liver disease.

- Sprouted brown rice decreases depression and fatigue in nursing mothers.

- Sprouted barley decreases blood pressure.

## Why Should Grains and Legumes Be Sprouted?

Think of grains like chicken eggs. There is a hard shell on the outside to protect the goodness on the inside. The shell is an obvious barrier to the nutrients inside. Most of our grains have a similar shell that contains an anti-nutrient called phytic acid, which acts like a barrier against the natural goodness inside the grain. Think of the elements in nature that the grain or seed must go through to be scattered onto the ground, dug down into the earth, and then sprout before it becomes a strong plant or vegetable. This barrier on the grain is natural protection. While this is good for the grains, preservation of the shell barrier is not so useful for our bodies—so we should soak or sprout the seeds, grains, and legumes before they are cooked or baked and eaten. When grains and seeds are soaked or sprouted, the natural hard shells becomes predigested and the phytic acid levels are lowered, allowing your body to absorb *more* of the nutrients available in the grain. If you have never tried sprouted or soaked seeds, grains, or legumes, I strongly encourage you to give them a try! Companies who manufacture sprouted or soaked grains are proud to display this healthy process that has been done for thousands of years (but recently forgotten with our demand for convenience foods). Sprouting and soaking takes time, but the benefits far outweigh the time it takes to produce *essential* nutrients.

### Seeds Are for More Than Just the Birds

Seeds like quinoa and Chia are high in fiber, antioxidants, and protein. Chia is also high in Omega-3s (see Chapter 7). Sprouted seeds are best. You can use seeds in:

- Yogurt
- Cereal
- Smoothies
- Salads
- Baked goods

The recommended serving size for most seeds is 1 tablespoon.

## Eating Against the Grain

The challenge of selecting carbs is eating against the grain (choosing whole, sprouted grains over processed, refined grains.) And the enjoyable part of my job is watching the transformation of those individuals who reduce their refined grain and sugar intake. Consuming less sugar has a sweet number of benefits:

- Less inflammation in the body—less pain in the muscles, joints, and bones (think about arthritis—which is inflammation in the joints)

- Weight loss—this one may seem obvious, but we often do not realize how much easier it is to lose weight until we reduce our sugar intake. I do not know how else to convince you but to beg you to reduce your consumption of added sugar and see the benefits for yourself. If you try nothing else with carbohydrate adjustments, try avoiding treats for a week and make informed choices with simple carbohydrates based on how you feel after that week.

- Reduces craving for sugar—over time (usually around two weeks), our bodies stop craving simple sugar and start craving and having more enjoyment of natural sugars in fruits and vegetables

- Healthy insulin response—your organs will be able to respond to the healthy sugars in fruits, vegetables, and dairy without getting worn out

The sugar count in the charts below excludes fruit, vegetable, and dairy sugars as these are found naturally in the food, rather than added to enhance flavor.

## You Have Options

### Breakfast

| Avoid this | Try this instead |
|---|---|
| Cereal and milk and lite mocha from coffee shop | 1 hardboiled egg, half of an orange, and green tea from coffee shop |
| Added sugar: *approximately 51 grams* | Added sugar: *zero grams* |

### Lunch

| Avoid this | Try this instead |
|---|---|
| White bread sandwich with deli meat, mayo, and 12 ounces soda | Salad with grilled chicken, avocado, cheese, nuts, and 20 ounces sparkling water |
| Added sugar: *approximately 56 grams* | Added sugar: *zero grams* |

### Dinner

| Avoid this | Try this instead |
|---|---|
| Restaurant burger, fries, and small shake | Restaurant veggie stir fry with lean beef or chicken and fresh fruit and cheese for dessert |
| Added sugar: *approximately 164 grams* | Added sugar: *zero grams* |

### Snack

| Avoid this | Try this instead |
|---|---|
| Gas station doughnut and chocolate milk | Gas station apple and string cheese stick |
| Added sugar: *approximately 104 grams* | Added sugar: *zero grams* |

*Daily total for "avoid this": 375 grams of added sugar or "try this": zero grams of added sugar.* The "avoid this" columns contain more than ten times the recommended daily total for added sugar. Let that fact settle for a moment.

## Are simple carbs the same as added sugars? **No.**

Simple carbs, like bleached, enriched flour pizza dough, probably contains little to no added sugar. However, due to the lack of nutrients in the enriched flour, the pizza dough has nearly the same effect on your body as added sugar.

If you cut out most added sugar and wonder why you still have severe sugar cravings, examine your simple carbohydrate intake.

*The less added sugars and simple carbs you consume, the less your body will crave. And you will have the added benefit of your body using fat as a main fuel source rather than mostly sugar (glucose).*

This sugar-filled day is a realistic tragedy for many Americans. "Avoid this" is what my day could have looked like over a decade ago when I consistently ate empty calories. I was tired and I had a stomachache all the time. Should we wonder why we suffer from so much chronic pain, obesity, and disease?

We must recognize the seriousness of our carbohydrate and sugar addiction. The mindset of "I have a sweet tooth and there is nothing I can do about my cravings" does not excuse preventable diseases. Sugar is killing us and addictions are getting worse with more and more convenience foods added to the market. *Now is the time to make changes in our thinking and in our actions.* Now is the time to be sick and tired of being sick and tired. How much longer are we willing to live with chronic pain, depression, anxiety, bottomless cravings, roller-coastering weight, daily fatigue, and disease?

You can do something about your health! You can take charge of your health! Small changes lead to a lifetime of healthier decisions. *You are the only one who can make the decision to become the person you were designed to be.* Will you make the commitment to try? Will you take steps to practice health?

*You can!*

Do you know how much added sugar you *need* per day to be healthy? If you guessed *zero grams*, you are correct.

**Trainer's Recommendation:** The American Heart Association recommends that men limit *added* sugar to 36 grams, or 9 teaspoons, per day and that women limit *added* sugar to 24 grams, or 6 teaspoons, per day. This does not include fruit, vegetable, and dairy sugar, which are balanced with nutrients, fiber, and no added sugars.

## Effect of Added Sugar on Children

Children are also negatively affected when consuming added sugar. Like adults, when children consume added sugar, their blood sugar rises and their little bodies produce insulin, which drives the blood sugar down too fast, causing:

- Brain fog

- Irritability

- Hunger headaches

- Sugar cravings

Knowing that I am cautious with added sugar and my own children, a few of my friends and family members try to sneak my children treats when they visit. I think about whether or not I am doing right by limiting sweets with added sugar. Am I depriving my children by not feeding and rewarding them with artificial, sugary treats? The answer is evident in their behavior. My children behave better when we say *no thank you* to the added sugar, artificial sugar, artificial color, and trans fats. Instead, we enjoy natural desserts like our favorite fruits, chemical-free ice cream and chocolate, and homemade treats sweetened with coconut, real cocoa, honey, and maple syrup. Saying a firm "no" to children when it comes to added sugar can be challenging at first (as adults, we know this struggle, right?), but "no" is the right word to say. Also, try phrases like:

- I am going to slice up some fresh strawberries for you instead.

- What is *your* favorite fruit? I will pick that up next time I am at the store.

- How about a square of dark chocolate instead? (And then be sure to put the rest *away*.)

Avoiding added sugar is especially important for children (and adults) with ADHD and autism. Because sugar affects our brain, the negative side effects are magnified for children with brain disorders.

*The more sugar we eat, the more we crave.* This cycle is true for children as well. Developing good habits with our families is challenging when everyone else gives in to the no-rules-apply attitude toward sugar. I challenge you to take the path less traveled and watch the benefits unfold. Like anything worthwhile, better health takes time and discipline. Practicing better choices will help keep brain health on the top of your priority list.

Summing up this monumental discovery, less added sugar equals less disease.

There are dozens of books on the shelves highlighting the dangerous effects of sugar. Yet the danger of sugar is such an unpopular topic. Is it because we are all addicted? Yes. We must reduce our sugar from simple carbs, packaged foods, processed foods, and sweets and increase our servings of fruits, vegetables, fat, and whole grains. Our lives depend on it. The quality of your life depends on it.

Reducing our sugar intake is that simple. Make small daily changes to reduce the amount of added sugar (without increasing artificial sweetener) you consume per day, and watch your energy increase as your waistline decreases. *Do not* be tricked into thinking you can

---

*I was amazed to learn that there is not one single function within my body that requires added sugar. Eat carrots, it will help your eyesight; eat spinach, it will boost your iron. Eat sugar and you will wreck everything you've tried so hard to fix.*

TRACY S.
ADVISORY BOARD MEMBER

### Are You Spoiling Your Children?

Whether you have children or not, you may interact with a child at some point. Do *not* think you are giving them a reward by constantly feeding them snacks and candy with added sugar. You are "spoiling" them—but not in the way you may be intending. Instead, offer your time and attention as a gift—this is what children treasure more than anything. Reserve "treats" for special occasions like birthdays and graduations.

swap sugar with artificial sweeteners to avoid the consequences. See Chapter 10 for more details.

## Practice

1. Practice reducing your number of added grams of sugar by half for the next three days and document how you feel.

_____

_____

How much more energy did you have toward the middle of day three?

_____

_____

Do you think you could cut down on sugar for a week? Yes/No

## Results:

2. Have you ever tried sprouted or soaked grains, seeds, or legumes?

_____

_____

_____

Try a new sprouted grain this week and record your experience:

_____

_____

_____

_____

_____

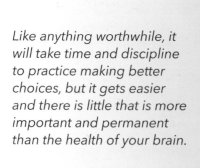

_Like anything worthwhile, it will take time and discipline to practice making better choices, but it gets easier and there is little that is more important and permanent than the health of your brain._

## S2L

Teach a friend the difference between sources of simple and complex carbohydrates.

Examine the dangerous affects of too much added sugar in our diets.

_____

_____

_____

Teach someone how much added sugar your body needs per day (_zero_, remember)

Who are you going to teach?

_____

**Additional Names for Refined, Added Sugar:**

- Dextrose
- Fructose
- Lactose
- Maltose
- Sucrose
- White sugar
- Corn syrup
- High fructose corn syrup
- Turbinado sugar

# InFIT Workout 6

First time (set) through: Warm up: Go through all of the exercises slowly, 15-20 repetitions each, with no resistance (no weight), 5-10 minutes. Second set: In the Strength Level, we continue performing all three exercises in each row before moving on to the next muscle group (Lower Body, Upper Body, and Core) with minimal rest in between exercises. Perform all nine exercises and then repeat as your fitness goals and time permit! This week we integrate more balance training, which is important for brain health, injury prevention, and a higher calorie burn. Remember to drink water during your workout and stretch tight muscles.

## Lower Body

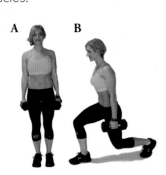

**DB Turning Lunge**

|  | Set 1 | Set 2 |
|---|---|---|
| Weight |  |  |
| Reps |  |  |

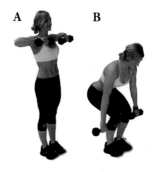

**DB Front Step Up to Balance**

|  | Set 1 | Set 2 |
|---|---|---|
| Weight |  |  |
| Reps |  |  |

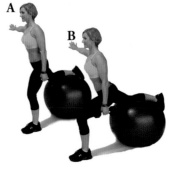

**DB SB Single Leg Lunge**

|  | Set 1 | Set 2 |
|---|---|---|
| Weight |  |  |
| Reps |  |  |

## Upper Body

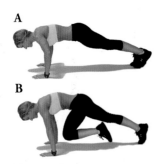

**Pushup ALT Knee In**

|  | Set 1 | Set 2 |
|---|---|---|
| Weight |  |  |
| Reps |  |  |

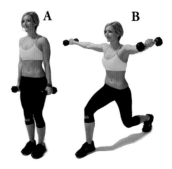

**DB Squat to Upright Row**

|  | Set 1 | Set 2 |
|---|---|---|
| Weight |  |  |
| Reps |  |  |

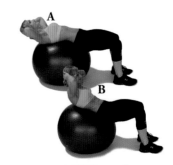

**DB Front Lunge to Lateral Raise**

|  | Set 1 | Set 2 |
|---|---|---|
| Weight |  |  |
| Reps |  |  |

## Core

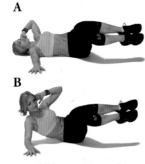

**Oblique Crunch**

|  | Set 1 | Set 2 |
|---|---|---|
| Weight |  |  |
| Reps |  |  |

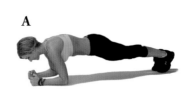

**Full Body Plank**

|  | Set 1 | Set 2 |
|---|---|---|
| Weight |  |  |
| Reps |  |  |

**SB Crunch**

|  | Set 1 | Set 2 |
|---|---|---|
| Weight |  |  |
| Reps |  |  |

# InFIT Workout 6–Option II

In the Strength Level, we continue performing all three exercises in each row before moving on to the next muscle group (Lower Body, Upper Body, and Core) with minimal rest in between exercises. Perform all nine exercises and then repeat as your fitness goals and time permit! This week we integrate more balance training, which is important for brain health, injury prevention, and a higher calorie burn. Remember to drink water during your workout and stretch tight muscles.

Lower Body

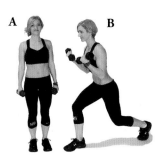

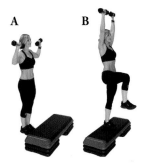

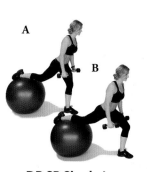

**DB Turning Lunge with Biceps Curl**

|  | Set 1 | Set 2 |
|---|---|---|
| **Weight** |  |  |
| **Reps** |  |  |

**DB Front Step Up to Balance with Shoulder Press**

|  | Set 1 | Set 2 |
|---|---|---|
| **Weight** |  |  |
| **Reps** |  |  |

**DB SB Single Leg Lunge Balance**

|  | Set 1 | Set 2 |
|---|---|---|
| **Weight** |  |  |
| **Reps** |  |  |

Upper Body

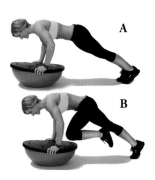

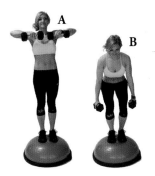

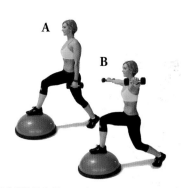

**BOSU Pushup ALT Knee In**

|  | Set 1 | Set 2 |
|---|---|---|
| **Weight** |  |  |
| **Reps** |  |  |

**BOSU DB Squat to Upright Row**

|  | Set 1 | Set 2 |
|---|---|---|
| **Weight** |  |  |
| **Reps** |  |  |

**BOSU DB Front Lunge to Lateral Raise**

|  | Set 1 | Set 2 |
|---|---|---|
| **Weight** |  |  |
| **Reps** |  |  |

Core

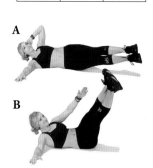

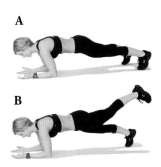

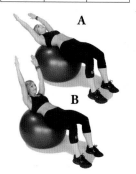

**Oblique Crunch–Straight Legs**

|  | Set 1 | Set 2 |
|---|---|---|
| **Weight** |  |  |
| **Reps** |  |  |

**Full Body Plank–ALT Single Leg**

|  | Set 1 | Set 2 |
|---|---|---|
| **Weight** |  |  |
| **Reps** |  |  |

**SB Crunch–Long Lever**

|  | Set 1 | Set 2 |
|---|---|---|
| **Weight** |  |  |
| **Reps** |  |  |

# ROAD MAP TO **SUCCESS**

## Review Your Map—Chapter Reflection

Use this road map as a weekly check-in to measure your goals and progress. Fill in the blank spaces at the bottom of the chart to create your own goals. The more often you check in with yourself, the more often you will bring health to the front of your mind, creating intention and success.

| | GOAL | MON Actual | TUE Actual | WED Actual | THU Actual | FRI Actual | SAT Actual | SUN Actual |
|---|---|---|---|---|---|---|---|---|
| Servings of produce (Ch 5) | | | | | | | | |
| Water in ounces | | | | | | | | |
| Hours of sleep (Ch 2) | | | | | | | | |
| Minutes of exercise | | | | | | | | |
| Weight | | | | | | | | |
| Amount of meals/ snacks per day (Ch 3) | | | | | | | | |
| Calories | | | | | | | | |
| Number of simple carbs (Ch 6) | | | | | | | | |
| Body fat % (optional) | | | | | | | | |
| Bowel movements (Ch 8) | | | | | | | | |
| **Add your own below** | | | | | | | | |
| | | | | | | | | |
| | | | | | | | | |
| | | | | | | | | |

Did you achieve most of your goals? _____ Why? _____

What is your plan for the next week to either stay on your original course or modify based on this week's review?

How do you feel about your progress thus far?

# LIVING AFFIRMATION
## WELLNESS FOR YOUR SOUL

## Unloading a Stressful Yoke

Come to Me, all you who labor and are heavy laden, and I will give you rest. Matthew 11:28

Due to our modern lifestyle and our consumptive pursuit of happiness, we are a stressed people. Symptoms of stress include burn out, depression, insomnia, weight struggles, and/or eating disorders. Stress can quickly develop into distress, as the felt urgencies and challenges of life become overwhelming. We learn from the Bible that God answers those who cry out to God, as David did in Psalm 20. Maybe you can testify to this truth as well.

*Are you in distress? Have you cried out to God? What is God saying to you?*

Jesus invites us to learn from him with these verses: "Come to Me, all *you* who labor and are heavy laden, and I will give you rest. Take My yoke upon you and learn from Me, for I am gentle and lowly in heart, and you will find rest for your souls. For My yoke is easy and My burden is light." Matthew 11:28-30

Allow the load of your life to change as you surrender your will to God's will. If you give God permission to replace or rearrange the priorities in your heart, you may be asked to let go of a few responsibilities, expectations, or even change course. As scary as this might seem, allow God to give you the rest that He has for you in His way. After all, God is the expert when it comes to resting assured.

Be blessed abundantly! ~ *Christina Zaczkowski*, MA, CPT

## *Reflection*

_____

_____

_____

# 7

# YOU CAN GET, OH, SATISFACTION!

## Principle Questions:

1. Does consuming dietary fat make you fat?

2. What are the four types of fat?

3. How much of your daily caloric intake should be from fat?

4. Why should you consume a balance of Omega-3 and Omega-6 fatty acids?

5. Why is cooking with certain oils dangerous?

6. Is it more expensive to eat clean?

**B**ecause healthy fat consumption is so satisfying, fat is one of my favorite topics in nutrition. It was probably one of my least favorites when I was overweight and unhealthy, but that is in my past and fat is a vital health topic, so let's examine fat together.

Consuming dietary fat does not make you fat. Dietary fat does not make you fat. No. Fat does not make you fat, and if you argue with me, you will see I am passionate to share the good news I have discovered. An *excess* of dietary fat can lead to the increase of body fat (adipose tissue). Guess what? The excess of *any* calorie, regardless where it comes from, leads to an increase in body fat. Remember, food is energy. If calories do not get used, they get stored!

Dietary fat plays a vital role in our brain and organ function, digestion, vitamin and mineral absorption, and nerve health. "But, Ashley, vital fat does not make me look better in my bathing suit," you might say. Our industrialized diets have been making a dangerous shift toward becoming a fat-free nation, based on the myth that eating fat makes us fat. This often leads to an increase in sodium, sugar, chemical additives, and/or refined grains in foods to make up for lost flavor and texture. Go back with me to high school biology. Which vitamins are fat-soluble? Right! A, D, E, and K. Tell me, has there been an equally rising correlation between the deficiency of vitamins A and D in our diets as they shift toward fat free? The answer is absolutely *yes* and the symptoms are evident.

Any extreme shift in nutrition on either side of excess or deficit is dangerous because our bodies were and are still designed for balance. Some fats are healthy in the proper proportions. Some are unhealthy altogether.

## Types of Fat

### Trans Fatty Acids (Trans Fats)

- Partially hydrogenated oils

### Saturated Fatty Acids (Saturated Fats)

- Animal fat: Eggs, butter, cheese, milk, and lard

- Tropical oils: Coconut and palm oil

### Monounsaturated Fatty Acids (Unsaturated Fats)

- Olive oil, nuts, vegetable oil, canola oil, high oleic safflower oil, sunflower oil, and avocados

**What to Look for in Oils**

Most processed oils become exposed to temperatures as high as 518 degrees Fahrenheit or more. High heat results in rancid oils. Rancid oils expose your body to free radicals known to cause heart disease and cancer, to name only a few problems. Once oils turn rancid in the refining process, they need to be bleached and deodorized. There is nothing natural about processed canola oil. Imagine spraying your salad with perfume or deodorant to make up for unpleasant, truth-revealing smells? The process of refining oils is a well kept, but tragic secret.

*Virgin and extra virgin oils are a safer alternative.* The process excludes extreme heat and toxic chemicals, making the oils safer to consume. Virgin oils are an essential investment into your health.

## Polyunsaturated Fatty Acids (Unsaturated Fats)

- Omega-3s: Fish oil, soybean oil, canola oil, walnuts, and flaxseed

- Omega-6s: Vegetable oils like safflower, corn, and soybean

# A Closer Look. Not All Fats Are Created Equal

# Avoid: *Trans*-Fatty Acids (Trans Fats)

We looked at trans fats in Chapter 2 when we talked about the dangers of partially hydrogenated oils in our foods. Partially hydrogenated oils are found in fried foods, packaged baked goods, processed snack foods (and most everything processed), margarines, et cetera. Yes, margarine. Am I telling you to get rid of margarine? No, I am asking nicely that you get rid of margarine. If you were eating it before, you probably thought margarine was a healthy alternative to butter. The Nurses' Health Study found that women who ate one and one-third tablespoons of margarine a day had a *50% greater risk of heart disease* than women who ate margarine only rarely. Alternatives to margarine include butter from organic, grass-fed cows; coconut oil; or extra virgin olive oil. How do you know if your favorite baked good contains trans fats? Read the label. If the ingredient list shows partially hydrogenated oils, put down the package and find a better alternative. I label most food ingredients as "better or worse," but when it comes to trans fats, they are just "bad." Make a point to stop eating trans fats and watch your health flourish. The fact that we came up with dozens of sugary ingredients to avoid, but only one type of fat to omit is interesting! We do *not* need to be scared of dietary fat. We need to be educated so we can make informed decisions. Udo Erasmus, PhD in nutrition, states the matter simply: "Trans fats bring twice as many food additives into our diet as all other food additives from all food sources combined."

## Saturated Fats

Saturated fats have a mixed review because so many people fear the alleged link to high cholesterol. Along with dietary fat, we do *not* need to fear cholesterol; the truth is that 999 people out of 1,000 can safely and effectively control their cholesterol with proper nutrition and exercise. Animal fats and saturated fats in tropical oils (in measured portions) offer wonderful health benefits and nutrients for your cells. Saturated fats also absorb essential vitamins. Experts suggest limiting saturated fats to no more than 10% of your daily calorie intake to avoid overexposure since saturated fats are found in every dietary fat and oil. Sources of healthy saturated fats to consume in moderation include eggs, milk, cheese, butter, lard, and tropical oils like coconut and palm oil. Cooking with and eating small amounts of tropical oils and animal fats have wonderful health properties, flavor, and satiating benefits.

## Mono- and Polyunsaturated Fats (Unsaturated Fats)

Mono and polyunsaturated fats play a vital role in maintaining optimal health as well. Unsaturated fats reduce inflammation, balance cholesterol levels, lower blood pressure, stabilize heart rhythms, and help stabilize blood sugar, which keeps your body feeling full and satisfied after a meal or snack. *Approximately 30-45% (some researchers even suggest up to 50%) of your daily calories should come from fat.* One of my favorite nutritionists and authors, Jonny Bowden, lists avocados (containing all three healthy sources of fat) as an outstanding choice for healthy fat in his book *The 150 Healthiest Foods on Earth.* Clients ask me if they should skip adding avocados or olive oil to their salads to cut calories. The answer every time is: *No,* do not compromise your health by skipping fats to make a calorie deficit. Instead, avoid refined grains, added sugar, and liquids (other than water) as a means of cutting unnecessary calories. Do you remember in Chapter 5 when we talked about eating a rainbow? Which vitamins are fat-soluble? Right again, A, D, E, and K. What does that mean? Fat-soluble means that you need to consume dietary fat for your body to break down and absorb the vitamins. If you are not getting enough healthy dietary fat, you are not absorbing vital nutrients.

When talking about polyunsaturated fat, we need to pause on Omega-3 and 6 fatty acids. Because we have moved away from a fish and vegetable meal profile, most Americans are severely lacking in Omega-3s. The consequences are evident. Unlike other nutrients, *our bodies do not produce omega fatty acids. Therefore, we need to obtain omegas through food and supplementation.* Omegas are vital for every function in your body. People who are active need even more omegas to help rebuild and repair cells that have been damaged during exercise. The key to unlocking benefits of omegas is not just *how much* you consume, the key is in the balance of Omega-3s to Omega-6s (between 1:1 and 1:4 servings, respectively).

## Omega-3 Fatty Acids (Omega-3s)

The federal government's latest dietary guidelines, released in 2011, suggest a specific amount for two main types of Omega-3s. To get a minimum daily intake of 250 milligrams of eicosapentaenoic acid (EPA) and docosahexaenoic acid (DHA), 8 ounces *per week* of any of the following combination of seafood is recommended. Below are some popular fish and shellfish and their approximate total content of EPA and DHA per 4 ounce portion:

- Salmon (Atlantic, Chinook, Coho): 1,200-2,400 milligrams

- Anchovies: 2,300-2,400 milligrams

> Unlike other nutrients, *our bodies do not produce omega fatty acids. Therefore, we need to obtain omegas through food and supplementation.*

### How Much Dietary Fat Do You Need?

Approximately 30-50% of your daily calories should come from fats.

This means that for a 1,200-calorie plan, you should consume about 40-67 grams of healthy fat per day.

For a 1,600-calorie plan, you should consume about 53-89 grams per day.

And for a 2,000-calorie plan, you should consume about 66-111 grams of fat per day.

If you did not calculate your approximate daily caloric intake, refer back to Chapter 1 for an estimate.

### Do You Need an Omega-3 Supplement?

If you do not eat fish at least one to two times per week, you may need an Omega-3 supplement; if so, look for one with at least 300 milligrams of DHA, vitamin E, or other stabilizer, and a source from small, oily fish like anchovy, sardines, or menhaden.

- Bluefin tuna: 1,700 milligrams; yellowfin tuna: 150-350 milligrams; canned: 150-300 milligrams

- Sardines: 1,100-1,600 milligrams

- Trout: 1,000-1,100 milligrams

- Crab: 200-550 milligrams

- Cod: 200 milligrams

- Scallops: 200 milligrams

- Lobsters: 200 milligrams

- Tilapia: 150 milligrams

- Shrimp: 100 milligrams

Non-fish sources of Omega-3s include flaxseed oil, beans, walnuts, seeds, and vegetables such as winter squash, broccoli, spinach, and cauliflower. Fish is the highest source of Omega-3s, but the danger of consuming too much (more than one to two times per week from polluted waters) may cause toxicity of heavy metals like mercury and lead in your body. Vegetable sources of Omega-3s are a great way to supplement your *daily* intake of Omega-3s.

## Omega-6 Fatty Acids (Omega-6s)

Omega-6s are more common in our diet than Omega-3s. Check the ingredient list of your favorite snack foods and you will likely find soybean oil and corn oil, two common sources of Omega-6s. We *do* need Omega-6s for our health; the proper amount helps reduce arthritis, allergies, ADHD, and even diabetes. But the problem is that *most of us get ten times more Omega-6s than we need* due to the heavy influence of soy and corn in our diets. By not getting enough Omega-3s and consuming too many Omega-6s, our body chemistry revolts (metabolic breakdown). An *excessive* amount of Omega-6s decreases your immune function, increases heart disease, and promotes unhealthy cell growth (leading to or exacerbating cancers). Are you starting to get the picture?

*We need more Omega-3s and fewer Omega-6s in our diets until we have cleaned up and kicked out the majority of packaged foods in our pantries.*

Eating a balance of Omega-3s and Omega-6s boosts your body's ability to fight off the common cold, complex diseases, and keeps lipids (fats) in check in your blood stream. Consuming a proper balance also leads to a reduction of inflammation in your body.

Remember Chapter 6? *Inflammation is the number one source of physical pain in your body and a breeding ground for disease.* The balance is especially important if you work out on a regular basis. Imagine pumping thick (full of fat) blood through a weak heart, clogged arteries, and swollen muscles: It looks like an aneurysm. Consuming the right amount of Omega-3s and Omega-6s (and practicing regular exercise) will keep your body pumping unclogged blood through a strong heart and healthy muscles.

There is an abundance of information on Omega-3s and -6s, so let me simplify by summarizing the recommendations of Erasmus:

- Eat one to two servings of wild-caught fish per week.

- Add a serving of flaxseed oil or walnuts to your meals or snacks three to four times per week.

- Eat vegetables like winter squash, broccoli, spinach, and cauliflower three to four times per week.

- Limit your foods containing corn and soy products to one or two servings per week *or less*. Always look for non-GMO soy and corn that has been minimally processed.

We have been chewing on beef jerky this chapter; it is thick stuff. The topic of dietary fat and its relationship to body fat has been so skewed over the past eighty years that this may be all new information. You know that balancing Omega-3s and Omega-6s is crucial in reducing chronic and acute inflammation, improving your immune system, and sharpening your brain. This chapter is fat with information! Here is the overview:

## What Are the Dangers of Not Getting *Enough* Healthy Dietary Fat?

- Damage to nerves

- Neurological problems (seizures in extreme cases)

- Problems with digestion and irregularity (bowel movements)

- Malnourishment of every cell in the body

- Feeling hungry all day long

- Chronic inflammation

- Low cholesterol

Has your doctor ever talked to you about triglyceride levels in your blood? Do not be too quick to point your finger at fat consumption. Consider the effect of added sugar on your body. When sugar is *not* burned off in your body, it turns into triglycerides in your blood stream. The excess triglycerides increase your risk of heart disease. High triglycerides are a result of eating too many refined sugars, not enough exercise, and not enough vitamins and minerals.

What is one thing you learned in this chapter?

Do you believe it?

What are some changes you will commit to in order to improve your dietary fat consumption?

Additional thoughts on the subject?

If you have not heard about the damaging effects of processed oils and the necessary effects of healthy dietary fat, ask a nutritionist or naturopath. If they have any current nutrition education, they will agree that processed oils are destructive and that dietary fat does not make you fat. An excess of calories makes you fat. *Furthermore*, not getting enough healthy fat has detrimental affects on your body.

- High blood pressure

- Exacerbation of degenerative diseases

## What Are the Dangers of Consuming *Trans* Fat?

- Inflammation in the body

- Cancer

- Weak immune system

- Heart disease

- Stroke

- Insulin resistance (diabetes)

## What Are the Benefits of *Balanced* Dietary Fat Intake?

- Properly absorb fat-soluble vitamins and minerals

- Nourish your brain

- Protect nerves

- Keep you satiated (feeling full) and avoid overeating

- Proper digestion

- Helps balance cholesterol

- Slows and reverses degenerative diseases

- Levels cholesterol and blood pressure

- Maintains healthy body weight

We are one of the best fed, poorly nourished nations in the world. Because of our busy lifestyles and sugar-accustomed taste buds, we have traded our health for convenience foods and sugar water, resulting in an upside-down health crisis. The state of health is looking dim, but you can make a difference for yourself right now with the foods you choose!

Remember, every meal and snack should include a healthy fat. Look back at all prior chapters in this book. Every *healthy* meal and snack idea includes *healthy* fat. Your body needs dietary fat!

Tip from Your Trainer: You can change your current eating habits if they need some improving. Change is hard, but many habits worth creating are challenging. Make small steps. Switch your fat-free dairy to 1% or more and exchange your margarine for organic butter. Include healthy fats and extra virgin oil on your salads and stir fries and commit to eating wild-caught fish one to two times per week.

**Cooking Tip from Your Trainer:** Use the guide below when cooking, baking, or frying your foods.

Low heat: Oils get damaged and carcinogenic when introduced to high heat. Instead, steam your veggies with water and drizzle the extra virgin oil on top before serving to preserve all of the nutrients.

Medium heat: Cooking with butter or tropical oils are good option when cooking over medium heat (for example, pan frying an egg or cooking 100% whole-grain, sprouted pasta).

High heat: For baking, grilling, or frying foods, use saturated fats such as lard, coconut, or palm oils. (For example, frying chicken or steak in coconut oil preserves the nutrients and gives the food a light, delicious flavor without the harmful effects of damaged oil.)

Learning and practicing how to use healthy fats to prepare and cook your foods not only removes a significant amount of carcinogens from your diet, but also offers rewarding benefits that will affect your health right now in tangible ways (*less pain in your joints* from inflammation, for instance).

## Practice

1. How much fat are you consuming per day? Track for three days and record it here:

Day 1  grams

Day 2  grams

Day 3  grams

2. How many servings of Omega-3s are you consuming per week? (Fish, flaxseeds, or walnuts)

3. Exercise. Did you know that consuming sugar without burning it off results in high triglycerides in your blood? Y/N

**Did You Know?**

The fat from healthy oils like fish and walnuts hold oxygen in our cells. Certain viruses, bacteria, fungi, and other foreign organisms cannot live in the presence of oxygen. Optimal consumption of healthy fat has tangible, positive effects on your immune system.

*Since adding extra virgin olive oil every day to my daughter's diet, she has attained a healthy body weight and her digestion has improved.*

DEBRA P.
INFIT CLIENT

## S2L

Explain the difference between healthy fats and unhealthy fats to a friend.

List examples of each type of fat. If you cannot remember, review the beginning of the chapter.

Also, educate someone who is very physically active on the benefits of balancing Omega-3s and Omega-6s. Also, let him or her know that among many other benefits, balancing omegas reduces inflammation (pain and soreness) and improves the immune system.

## Fat-Friendly Day—Example Ideas

## Breakfast:

- Organic whole milk in your coffee
- Organic 1/2 tablespoon butter on sprouted wheat bread
- One pan-fried egg with Swiss cheese
- 1/2 of an orange

## Mid-morning Snack:

- One banana with a handful of raw or soaked, unsalted nuts (almonds, cashews, and walnuts)
- One apple with almond butter or string cheese

## Lunch:

- Salad with organic dressing (avoid trans fats) or extra virgin oil/balsamic vinegar and seasoning
- 1/2 of a small avocado
- Protein—chicken or fish (on the side or on your salad)

## Mid-day Snack:

- Homemade fruit smoothie with one serving of all natural heavy whipping cream or plain Greek yogurt

## Dinner:

- Grilled or baked burgers or steak

- Variety of steamed vegetables with extra virgin olive or hemp oil

## Dessert:

- A glass of coconut or almond milk and one square of dark chocolate

## Seasoning Mix Idea (homemade—use within three days):

- Oregano, dill, basil, fresh lemon, unsweetened coconut flakes, Celtic sea salt, and pepper. Mix together and drizzle on veggies, salad, or pasta.

**Hemp oil** is a delicious source of Omega-3s and 6s. This flavorful oil is great in soups, salads, dressings, and stir frys.

# InFIT Workout 7

First time (set) through: Warm up: Go through all of the exercises slowly, 15-20 repetitions each, with no resistance (no weight), 5-10 minutes. Second set: In the Strength Level, we continue performing all three exercises in each row before moving on to the next muscle group (Lower Body, Upper Body, and Core) with minimal rest in between exercises. Perform all nine exercises and then repeat as your fitness goals and time permit! Core stabilization is emphasized in InFIT Workout 7. Nearly every exercise in this workout includes a component of core training to continue toning and strengthening your midsection. Remember to drink water during your workout and stretch tight muscles.

## Lower Body

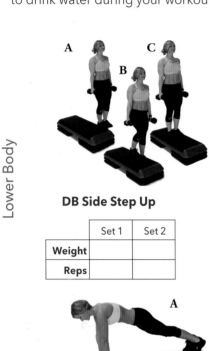

**DB Side Step Up**

|  | Set 1 | Set 2 |
|---|---|---|
| Weight |  |  |
| Reps |  |  |

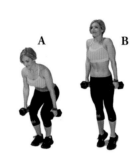

**DB Squat to Toes**

|  | Set 1 | Set 2 |
|---|---|---|
| Weight |  |  |
| Reps |  |  |

**DB Deadlift**

|  | Set 1 | Set 2 |
|---|---|---|
| Weight |  |  |
| Reps |  |  |

## Upper Body

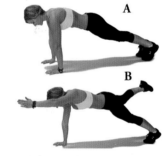

**Plank with ALT Arm/Leg Extension**

|  | Set 1 | Set 2 |
|---|---|---|
| Weight |  |  |
| Reps |  |  |

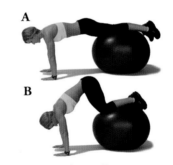

**SB Pike Roll Up**

|  | Set 1 | Set 2 |
|---|---|---|
| Weight |  |  |
| Reps |  |  |

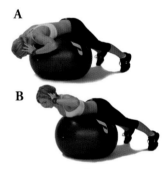

**SB Back Extension**

|  | Set 1 | Set 2 |
|---|---|---|
| Weight |  |  |
| Reps |  |  |

## Core

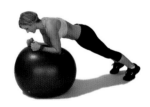

**SB Plank**

|  | Set 1 | Set 2 |
|---|---|---|
| Weight |  |  |
| Reps |  |  |

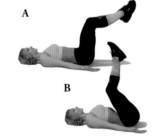

**Reverse Crunch**

|  | Set 1 | Set 2 |
|---|---|---|
| Weight |  |  |
| Reps |  |  |

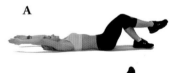

**Single Leg Lift**

|  | Set 1 | Set 2 |
|---|---|---|
| Weight |  |  |
| Reps |  |  |

# InFIT Workout 7–Option II

In the Strength Level, we continue performing all three exercises in each row before moving on to the next muscle group (Lower Body, Upper Body, and Core) with minimal rest in between exercises. Perform all nine exercises and then repeat as your fitness goals and time permit! Core stabilization is emphasized in InFIT Workout 7. Nearly every exercise in this workout includes a component of core training to continue toning and strengthening your midsection. Remember to drink water during your workout and stretch tight muscles.

Lower Body

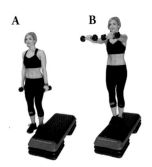

**DB Side Step Up with Front Raise**

|         | Set 1 | Set 2 |
|---------|-------|-------|
| Weight  |       |       |
| Reps    |       |       |

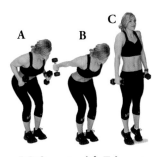

**DB Squat with Triceps Kickback Shrug to Toes**

|         | Set 1 | Set 2 |
|---------|-------|-------|
| Weight  |       |       |
| Reps    |       |       |

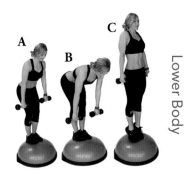

**DB BOSU Deadlift with Shrug**

|         | Set 1 | Set 2 |
|---------|-------|-------|
| Weight  |       |       |
| Reps    |       |       |

Upper Body

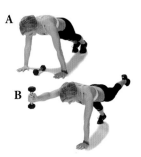

**DB Plank with ALT Arm/Leg Extension**

|         | Set 1 | Set 2 |
|---------|-------|-------|
| Weight  |       |       |
| Reps    |       |       |

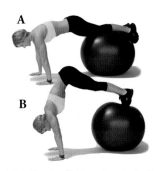

**SB Pike Roll Up–Straight Leg**

|         | Set 1 | Set 2 |
|---------|-------|-------|
| Weight  |       |       |
| Reps    |       |       |

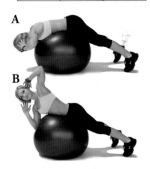

**SB Back Extension with Rotation**

|         | Set 1 | Set 2 |
|---------|-------|-------|
| Weight  |       |       |
| Reps    |       |       |

Core

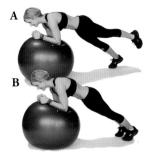

**SB Plank–Single Leg**

|         | Set 1 | Set 2 |
|---------|-------|-------|
| Weight  |       |       |
| Reps    |       |       |

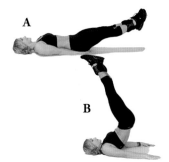

**Reverse Crunch–Add Ankle Weights**

|         | Set 1 | Set 2 |
|---------|-------|-------|
| Weight  |       |       |
| Reps    |       |       |

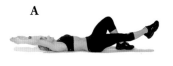
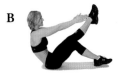

**Single Leg Lift–Straight Leg**

|         | Set 1 | Set 2 |
|---------|-------|-------|
| Weight  |       |       |
| Reps    |       |       |

# ROAD MAP TO **SUCCESS**

## Review Your Map—Chapter Reflection

Use this road map as a weekly check-in to measure your goals and progress. Fill in the blank spaces at the bottom of the chart to create your own goals. The more often you check in with yourself, the more often you will bring health to the front of your mind, creating intention and success.

| | GOAL | MON | TUE | WED | THU | FRI | SAT | SUN |
|---|---|---|---|---|---|---|---|---|
| | | Actual | Actual | Actual | Actual | Actual | Actual | Actual |
| Servings of produce (Ch 5) | | | | | | | | |
| Water in ounces | | | | | | | | |
| Hours of sleep (Ch 2) | | | | | | | | |
| Minutes of exercise | | | | | | | | |
| Weight | | | | | | | | |
| Amount of meals/ snacks per day (Ch 3) | | | | | | | | |
| Calories | | | | | | | | |
| Number of simple carbs (Ch 6) | | | | | | | | |
| Body fat % (optional) | | | | | | | | |
| Bowel movements (Ch 8) | | | | | | | | |
| **Add your own below** | | | | | | | | |
| | | | | | | | | |
| | | | | | | | | |
| | | | | | | | | |

Did you achieve most of your goals? _____ Why? _____

What is your plan for the next week to either stay on your original course or modify based on this week's review?

How do you feel about your progress thus far?

# LIVING AFFIRMATION
## WELLNESS FOR YOUR SOUL

## Good News, My Friend!

Then Jesus said to those Jews who believed Him, "If you abide in My word, you are My disciples indeed. And you shall know the truth, and the truth shall make you free." John 8:31-32

*Living Wellness* is not about getting healthier or losing weight by following a set of rules. Sometimes, when we are handed rules, our natural response is to challenge them. *Living Wellness* helps you discover the truth about health, fitness, and wellness by taking small, but consistent steps to improve your life. Truth offers freedom.

Here is another hard truth about our nutrition: How can we honestly say that foods containing trans fats are so delicious when the long-term effects of having them are so dangerous? We know better now and, by choosing truth rather than following a list of rules for our nutritional health, we are taking responsibility, which changes everything. Without understanding, good nutrition remains nothing but a set of rules.

*After reading this chapter, do you feel relieved with the truth that consuming healthy dietary fat is vital to life and that it does not contradict weight loss?*

*In what aspects of your life do you feel as though you are following a set of rules without understanding why?*

Prayerfully ponder what God has to say about freedom through truth.

Be blessed abundantly! ~ *Christina Zaczkowski, MA, CPT*

## *Reflection*

_____

_____

_____

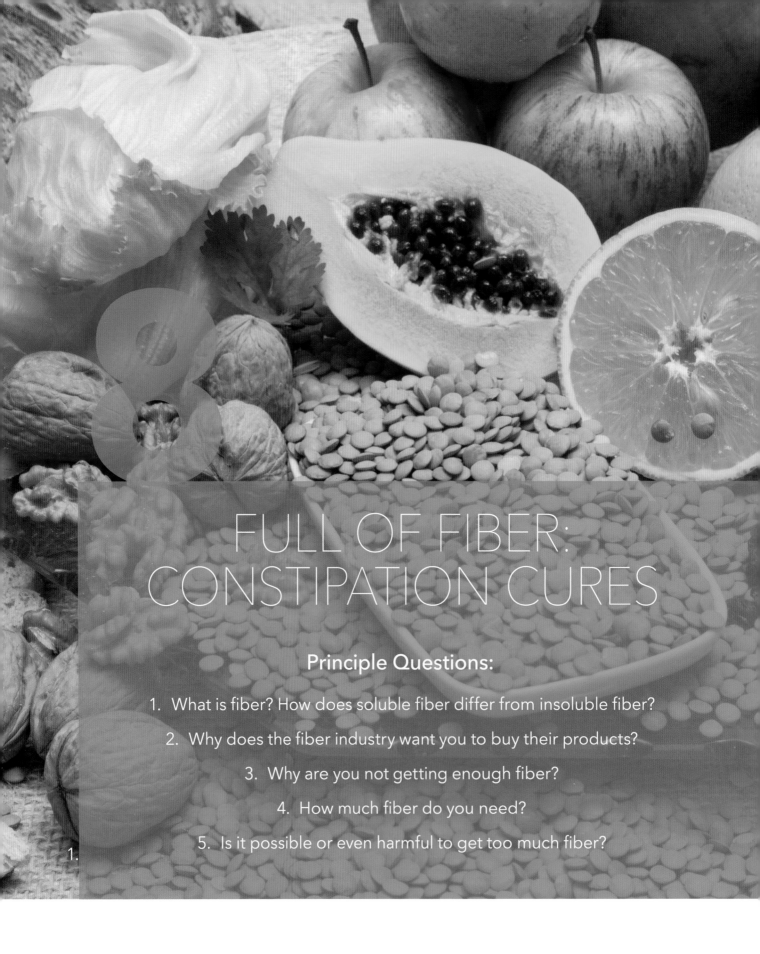

# FULL OF FIBER:
# CONSTIPATION CURES

### Principle Questions:

1. What is fiber? How does soluble fiber differ from insoluble fiber?

2. Why does the fiber industry want you to buy their products?

3. Why are you not getting enough fiber?

4. How much fiber do you need?

5. Is it possible or even harmful to get too much fiber?

1.

Along with fat, fiber is another touchy topic (and a billion-dollar industry). Fiber One, Fiber Plus, Fibertastic, Fiberific, Fiberlicious—every fiber-like food product has been manufactured in the last decade, and do you know why? Not because we all woke up and decided we need more fiber, but because we are all constipated.

There. I said we are constipated. It is a fact.

Look at what we are eating and you will find the answer as to *why*: PPC.

- Packaged
- Processed
- Convenience

There is no fiber in that combination. No real fiber, that is. *If we consumed the recommended amount of fruits, veggies, and water per day, the fiber industry would crash overnight.* I do not wish this upon any industry, but I would like to see us eating more fiber organically.

## What Is Fiber?

Dietary fiber, also known as roughage or bulk, includes all parts of plant foods that your body does not digest or absorb (Sounds pleasing to eat, right?). Fiber is like a magnet or a sponge floating through your digestive tract. While protein, carbs, and fat break down and absorb in your body, fiber stays intact and attracts toxins that need to be eliminated from your body.

## Sponges and Magnets

### Soluble Fiber

Soluble fiber dissolves in water to form a sponge-like substance. This type of fiber is responsible for balancing cholesterol and blood sugar levels (think back in Chapter 6 about what makes some carbs turn into sugar quickly and other carbs keep your blood sugar stable). Soluble fiber is found in, but not limited to the following:

- Apples
- Barley
- Beans
- Carrots
- Citrus fruits
- Oats
- Peas
- Psyllium

**Benefits of Fiber:**

- Balances cholesterol
- Lowers blood sugar levels
- Gathers toxins and eliminates them through the digestive system
- Regulates bowel movements
- Helps keep your weight in check by keeping you full after meals and snacks

Still constipated? Do you take medication? If you are eating the recommended fruits, vegetables, and fiber per day and you are still constipated, check your medication symptoms and side effects. Some medications cause constipation. Ask your doctor for the most natural remedies available.

## Insoluble Fiber

Insoluble fiber is like a magnet that increases stool bulk and promotes the movement of material through your digestive system. It also helps you feel full after meals and snacks. This type of fiber benefits individuals who struggle with constipation or irregular stools. Insoluble fiber is found in but not limited to these foods:

- Beans
- Green beans
- Potatoes
- Whole wheat flour
- Cauliflower
- Nuts
- Wheat bran

Soluble fiber absorbs toxic material and waste from your body like a sponge and insoluble fiber attracts the toxic material like a magnet through the intestines, providing a healthy cleansing for your colon every day.

Instead of relying on bars and shakes, which are usually loaded with added sugar and preservatives, most of your fiber should be from raw fruits, raw and steamed veggies, whole grains, and beans. Consuming a variety of sources offers an important balance of soluble and insoluble fiber.

What natural sources of fiber do you like?

Take an honest look at what you eat all day.

Do you naturally avoid foods that are high in fiber? Yes/No

Why?

*"The opposite of love is not hate, it's indifference. The opposite of beauty is not ugliness, it's indifference. The opposite of faith is not heresy, it's indifference. And the opposite of life is not death, but indifference between life and death."*

ELIE WIESEL

## How Much Fiber Do You Need?

### Trainer's Recommendation (Mayo Clinic):

|  | Age 50 or younger | Age 51 or older |
|---|---|---|
| **Men** | 38 grams | 30 grams |
| **Women** | 25 grams | 21 grams |

So, how much fiber do *you* need per day? _____ grams

## Fiber-Rich Foods

- Fruits (a minimum of two to three servings per day is recommended)—see Chapter 5 for a complete list

- Vegetables (a minimum of two to three servings per day is recommended)—see Chapter 5 for a complete list

- Whole grains (two to three servings per day is recommended—sprouted when available)—see Chapter 6 for a complete list of whole grains

- Legumes (one serving per day of either lentils or beans)

We would get plenty of fiber if we consumed the recommended amount of each of the above categories. Yet, I often hear that eating healthy is too expensive. How much do fiber supplements cost? How much do diet programs cost? How much do doctor visits cost for digestive problems, chronic illnesses, and preventable diseases? I am not judging your habits. I, too, have struggled with regular intestinal movements in the past, but it is so refreshing to know that you can be in control of your body. You make choices every day that affect your health. Make decisions for better health, the raw and organic way.

**Tip from Your Trainer:**
Instead of grabbing a fiber bar, try combining 1/4 cup of blueberries, 2 tablespoons of walnuts, and 1 tablespoon of natural, dark chocolate chips. The combination is packed with fiber, antioxidants, and healthy fat. Perfect for an energy boost and digestive aid!

## Do You Need a Fiber Supplement?

If you are still constipated after consuming the recommended fruits, veggies, and beans, there are a few other avenues to explore before you take a fiber supplement—not because they are necessarily bad, but because you may be missing the root cause of the problem.

## Constipation Troubleshooting

- Try more raw fruits and vegetables—Leave the skin on when appropriate and take your time to chew your food (try lightly cooked if have a hard time digesting raw veggies).

- Water—Are you still drinking half of your ideal body weight in ounces of water? If not, start now. Remember, soluble fiber needs water to turn it into a sponge, absorbing and eliminating toxins from your body.

- Healthy fat—Consuming healthy dietary fats aid in digestion. Try adding 1 tablespoon of extra virgin oil to your salad and another to your steamed vegetables (every day) for improved regularity. Refer to Chapter 7 for a complete list of healthy fats.

- Move more—Your digestive system needs to be exercised just as much as your heart and muscles. Exercise will help the intestines get the bowels moving, from the inside out.

If none of the troubleshooting ideas work and you still want a fiber supplement, look for one with the least amount of additives and sugar. A Nutrition Response Testing physician may help find an unresolved problem with your digestion.

## Too Much of a Good Thing?

Getting too much fiber has adverse effects: loose stools, abdominal discomfort, gas, bloating, and intestinal blockage. Fibers such as guar gum, inulin, oligofructose, polydextrose, psyllium, and starch have been found to cause abdominal cramping, bloating, gas, and diarrhea—especially when taken in excess.

Also, remember that fiber acts like a magnet for toxins. Too much fiber also acts like a *magnet to minerals* such as iron, zinc, calcium, and magnesium, and can decrease their absorption in your digestive tract. We need those nutrients! Let's not work *against* our bodies by getting too much of a good thing.

*My smile is one of the most powerful forces on earth. Others will wonder at the source of your smile as you experience joy resulting from the struggle and perseverance to become the whole person God created you to be, physically, mentally, and spiritually.*

JULIE F.
INFIT CORPORATE
PROMOTIONS CONSULTANT

### S2L

Do not skip this part!

Discuss the benefits of fiber (see the chart at the beginning of this chapter for specifics) with a friend or mature adult (remember, mature adults need slightly less fiber than child-bearing age adults).

Who are you going to share this with?

Describe an adequate amount of fiber (grams per day) and what sources are good options.

## Just the Right Amount

Usually when you begin eliminating ingredients like added sugar, simple carbs, and trans fats from your diet and replacing them with healthy produce, protein, and fat, you lose several pounds within the first week due to elimination. Think about how much food you consume in a day, a week, or a month. If you simply consume less or digest your food with more efficiency, you will lighten up instantly. Eating the right amount of fiber from whole foods assists in your healthy weight and keeps your body detoxified without the need for expensive and complicated cleanses. Natural fiber saves you money!

## High-Fiber Bean Beef Burgers

*Serves 6*

1 cup filtered water

1/2 cup bulgur

1 can (15 ounces) black beans, rinsed and drained (preferably soaked overnight)

3 green onions, sliced

1 tablespoon stone-ground mustard

1 garlic clove, halved

1/4 teaspoon mineral salt

1/4 teaspoon pepper

1 egg, lightly beaten

1/2 pound lean grass-fed ground beef (90% lean)

1 tablespoon extra virgin olive oil

6 100% sprouted grain hamburger buns, split

Spinach leaves, sliced red onion, and tomato

### Directions

In a small saucepan, bring water to a boil. Stir in bulgur. Reduce heat; cover and simmer for 15-20 minutes or until tender. In a food processor, combine the beans, onions, mustard, and garlic. Cover and pulse until blended. Stir in salt and pepper.

In a large bowl, combine the egg, bulgur, and bean mixture. Crumble beef over mixture and mix well. Shape into six patties.

In a large nonstick skillet, cook patties in oil in batches for four to five minutes on each side or until a meat thermometer reads 160 degrees Fahrenheit and juices run clear. Serve on a sprouted grain bun with spinach, onion, and tomato.

## Nutritional Facts

1 burger (calculated without spinach, onion and tomato) equals 307 calories, 8 grams of fat (2 grams saturated fat), 54 milligrams cholesterol, 517 milligrams sodium, 42 grams carbohydrate, 9 grams fiber, 17 grams protein. Diabetic Exchanges: 2 starch, 2 lean meat, 1 fat.

Originally published as Bean Beef Burgers in *Healthy Cooking* February/March 2010.

# Review

What is the difference between soluble and insoluble fiber? (Think sponge versus magnet)

How much fiber do you need? _____ grams per day

Is there harm in getting too much fiber?

Why?

What are the benefits of fiber?

Are you taking a fiber supplement? Why?

After reading this chapter, do you still feel as though you need to supplement your fiber intake?

# Practice

1. Track your fiber intake for three days and record it here:

   Day 1  grams _____

   Day 2  grams _____

   Day 3  grams _____

2. What are some of your favorite sources of fiber?

   _____

3. How can you get more fiber from food in your day?

   _____

4. Do you have any additional thoughts on this subject?

   _____

# InFIT Workout 8

First time (set) through: Warm up: Go through all of the exercises slowly, 15-20 repetitions each, with no resistance (no weight), 5-10 minutes. Second set: In the Strength Level, we continue performing all three exercises in each row before moving on to the next muscle group (Lower Body, Upper Body, and Core) with minimal rest in between exercises. Perform all nine exercises and then repeat as your fitness goals and time permit! Remember to drink water during your workout and stretch tight muscles.

**Lower Body**

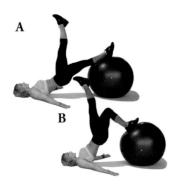

**SB Hamstring Curl–Single Leg**

|  | Set 1 | Set 2 |
|---|---|---|
| **Weight** | | |
| **Reps** | | |

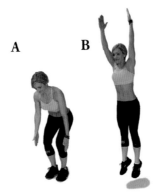

**Squat Jump**

|  | Set 1 | Set 2 |
|---|---|---|
| **Weight** | | |
| **Reps** | | |

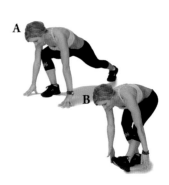

**Runner's Start to Lunge**

|  | Set 1 | Set 2 |
|---|---|---|
| **Weight** | | |
| **Reps** | | |

**Upper Body**

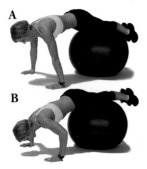

**SB Pushup**

|  | Set 1 | Set 2 |
|---|---|---|
| **Weight** | | |
| **Reps** | | |

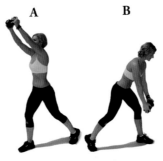

**DB Chop**

|  | Set 1 | Set 2 |
|---|---|---|
| **Weight** | | |
| **Reps** | | |

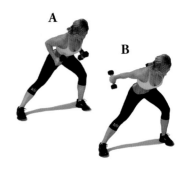

**DB Lateral Lunge with Triceps Kickback**

|  | Set 1 | Set 2 |
|---|---|---|
| **Weight** | | |
| **Reps** | | |

**Core**

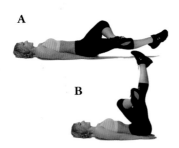

**Cross Leg Crunch with Straight Legs**

|  | Set 1 | Set 2 |
|---|---|---|
| **Weight** | | |
| **Reps** | | |

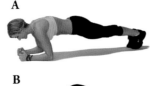
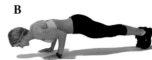

**Plank to Triceps Pushup**

|  | Set 1 | Set 2 |
|---|---|---|
| **Weight** | | |
| **Reps** | | |

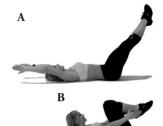

**Pilates Double Leg Stretch**

|  | Set 1 | Set 2 |
|---|---|---|
| **Weight** | | |
| **Reps** | | |

# InFIT Workout 8—Option II

In the Strength Level, we continue performing all three exercises in each row before moving on to the next muscle group (Lower Body, Upper Body, and Core) with minimal rest in between exercises. Perform all nine exercises and then repeat as your fitness goals and time permit! Remember to drink water during your workout and stretch tight muscles.

## Lower Body

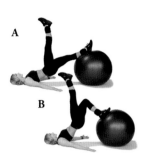

### SB Hamstring Curl–Single Leg with Ankle Weights

|         | Set 1 | Set 2 |
|---------|-------|-------|
| Weight  |       |       |
| Reps    |       |       |

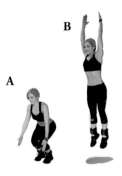

### Squat Jump with Ankle Weights

|         | Set 1 | Set 2 |
|---------|-------|-------|
| Weight  |       |       |
| Reps    |       |       |

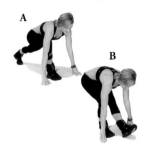

### Runner's Start to Lunge with Ankle Weights

|         | Set 1 | Set 2 |
|---------|-------|-------|
| Weight  |       |       |
| Reps    |       |       |

## Upper Body

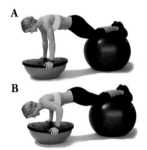

### BOSU SB Pushup

|         | Set 1 | Set 2 |
|---------|-------|-------|
| Weight  |       |       |
| Reps    |       |       |

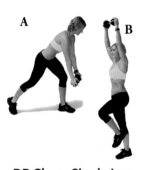

### DB Chop–Single Leg

|         | Set 1 | Set 2 |
|---------|-------|-------|
| Weight  |       |       |
| Reps    |       |       |

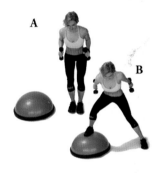

### BOSU DB Lateral Lunge with Triceps Kickback

|         | Set 1 | Set 2 |
|---------|-------|-------|
| Weight  |       |       |
| Reps    |       |       |

## Core

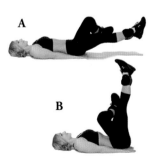

### Cross Leg Crunch–Straight Legs–Add Ankle Weights

|         | Set 1 | Set 2 |
|---------|-------|-------|
| Weight  |       |       |
| Reps    |       |       |

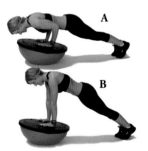

### BOSU Triceps Pushup

|         | Set 1 | Set 2 |
|---------|-------|-------|
| Weight  |       |       |
| Reps    |       |       |

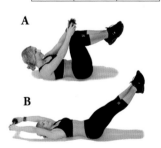

### DB Pilates Double Leg Stretch

|         | Set 1 | Set 2 |
|---------|-------|-------|
| Weight  |       |       |
| Reps    |       |       |

# ROAD MAP TO **SUCCESS**

## Review Your Map—Chapter Reflection

Use this road map as a weekly check-in to measure your goals and progress. Fill in the blank spaces at the bottom of the chart to create your own goals. The more often you check in with yourself, the more often you will bring health to the front of your mind, creating intention and success.

| | GOAL | MON Actual | TUE Actual | WED Actual | THU Actual | FRI Actual | SAT Actual | SUN Actual |
|---|---|---|---|---|---|---|---|---|
| **Servings of produce (Ch 5)** | | | | | | | | |
| **Water in ounces** | | | | | | | | |
| **Hours of sleep (Ch 2)** | | | | | | | | |
| **Minutes of exercise** | | | | | | | | |
| **Weight** | | | | | | | | |
| **Amount of meals/ snacks per day (Ch 3)** | | | | | | | | |
| **Calories** | | | | | | | | |
| **Number of simple carbs (Ch 6)** | | | | | | | | |
| **Body fat % (optional)** | | | | | | | | |
| **Bowel movements (Ch 8)** | | | | | | | | |
| **Add your own below** | | | | | | | | |
| | | | | | | | | |
| | | | | | | | | |
| | | | | | | | | |

Did you achieve most of your goals? _____ Why? _____

What is your plan for the next week to either stay on your original course or modify based on this week's review?

How do you feel about your progress thus far?

# LIVING AFFIRMATION
## WELLNESS FOR YOUR SOUL

## The Forgiveness Fiber

So He said to them, "Are you thus without understanding also? Do you not perceive that whatever enters a man from outside cannot defile him, because it does not enter his heart but his stomach, and is eliminated, thus purifying all foods?" (In saying this, Jesus declared all foods clean.) Mark 7:18-19

Let me give you the context of these verses: After admonishing the tradition-loving and law-loving Pharisees, Jesus explains to his disciples that they can go through all the motions of attempting to be righteous in God's sight, but completely miss righteousness if their hearts are not honest. Jesus uses a picture we can all relate to: food. We eat, which passes through us, and eventually leaves us. Food does not make us unclean in a spiritual sense; our very own heart may be the root problem. In the scripture verse, Jesus tells the Pharisees that God does not care for religious acts. God cares for a dedicated heart.

*How does Jesus' example of food relate to our spiritual state?*

If the food we ingest contains no fiber, our bodies hang on to what we ate and it rots in our gut. If our heart's attitude lacks the fiber of forgiveness, and we hang on to offenses committed against us, that lack of forgiveness will make us rot in the soul and in the body. Forgiveness is one of the main themes in Christianity, making everyone equal to the need for forgiveness. We all need God's forgiveness and the forgiveness of one another.

*Do you need to forgive someone?* Ask God to help you forgive.

Fiber is comparable to forgiveness: We need both to be clean—in our gut and in our heart. I invite you to prayerfully do an inventory of your heart. Jesus shows us how by becoming the way to peace with God and peace with each other. We are called to forgive one another as God has forgiven us. "To forgive is to set a prisoner free and discover that the prisoner was you." – Lewis B. Smedes

Be blessed abundantly! ~ *Christina Zaczkowski*, MA, CPT

## *Reflection*

_____

_____

_____

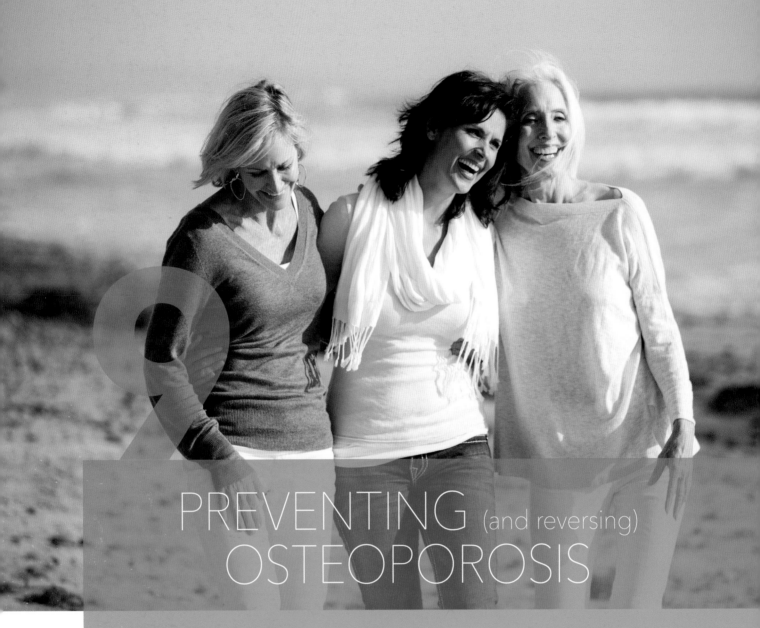

# PREVENTING (and reversing) OSTEOPOROSIS

## Principle Questions:

1. What is osteoporosis and osteoarthritis? Who is at risk?

2. What are the controllable and uncontrollable risk factors surrounding osteoporosis?

3. Why is it important to get enough (but not too much) vitamin D with calcium?

4. What are synthetic vitamins?

5. How does strength training improve your bone density?

As we age, we often think that breaking bones and wearing cartilage is just a normal part of growing old. The reality is that we do not have to lose all of our bone density and soft tissue, but it takes intentional action to keep our muscles and bones strong and healthy.

**Osteoporosis** is a result of bone loss and/or the body ceasing to make bone tissue. The National Osteoporosis Foundation (NOF) states: "About 10 million Americans have osteoporosis. About 34 million are at risk for the disease. Estimates suggest that about half of all women older than 50, and up to one in four men, will break a bone because of osteoporosis."

**Osteoarthritis** is a similar condition that results from worn-down cartilage that covers the ends of bones at a joint. Osteoarthritis causes joint pain and reduced range of motion.

Osteoporosis and osteoarthritis affect both men and women, but women are more at risk for the diseases. The conditions are more common in mature adults. They are expensive and debilitating diseases. Osteoporosis and osteoarthritis are not inevitable with aging. We can protect our bones and soft tissue at all stages of life. According to the NOF, there are uncontrollable and controllable risk factors that should be considered with osteoporosis.

## Uncontrollable Risk Factors (NOF)

- Being over age 50
- Being female
- Menopause
- Family history
- Low body weight and/or being small and thin
- Broken bones or height loss

## Controllable Risk Factors (NOF)

- Not getting enough calcium and vitamin D
- Not eating enough fruits and vegetables
- Getting too much sodium and caffeine
- Having an inactive lifestyle
- Smoking
- Drinking too much alcohol

*The number one thing that keeps me motivated to take care of myself is my three beautiful girls. They (we all) need exercise, sleep, and healthy foods to be the best we can be at whatever we are doing—I want to model these behaviors so that my girls have the knowledge and confidence to make healthy choices for the rest of their lives!*

Jill M.
InFIT PT Manager

*A merry heart does good, like medicine, But a broken spirit dries the bones.*

PROVERBS *17:22*

*My solid body and strong bones are a result of my nutrition and physical activity growing up on a dairy farm. Fresh, organic whole milk and my daily physical lifestyle laid the foundation for my strong body. Now I keep myself healthy by limiting sugar, eating plenty of fruits and vegetables, and exercising my body as often as I can.*

Donna S.
InFIT client

*Let food be thy medicine and medicine be thy food.*
Hippocrates

- Being overweight

**Below are four main ways to prevent and lessen the symptoms of osteoporosis and osteoarthritis:**

1. Balanced nutrition

2. Resistance training

3. Avoiding smoking

4. Limiting alcohol

## Balanced Nutrition—Calcium, Magnesium, Vitamin D

We all know that calcium is good for maintaining strong bones. The National Academy of Sciences currently recommends that people ages 19 to 50 consume 1,000 milligrams of calcium per day, and that those age 50 or over get 1,200 milligrams per day.

*It takes a variety of only two to three servings of dairy, almond milk, or coconut milk per day to reach 1,200 milligrams per day.* If you are lactose sensitive and do not consume dairy, you can incorporate a variety of vegetables, fruits, nuts, and seeds to make up the difference.

## Good Sources of Calcium

- Blackstrap molasses

- Collards, bok choy, baked beans, and natural supplements that contain both calcium and vitamin D

- Organic milk, yogurt, cheese, eggs, and other dairy

- Nuts like almonds and Brazil nuts

- Oranges

- Sesame seeds

- Vegetables like okra, spinach, kelp, broccoli, and celery

## Too Much of a Good Thing?

What most people do not know is that too much calcium, by itself, can be harmful. Research indicates that too much calcium (an excess of 1,200 milligrams in women and 2,000 milligrams in men) has been linked with ovarian and prostate cancers. It is important to consume calcium from a wide variety of sources, and it is best to combine it with foods containing vitamin D and magnesium for optimal absorption.

## Vitamin D

Calcium *without* vitamin D leads to a possible *decrease* in absorption in your body. In addition to maintaining strong bones, vitamin D also has these benefits:

- Prevents autoimmune diseases

- Prevents several types of cancers

- Reduces the risk of cardiovascular disease

### How Much Vitamin D Do You Need?

| Women and Men | |
|---|---|
| **Under age 50** | **Age 50 and older** |
| 400-800 international units (IU) daily* | 800-1,000 IU daily* |

*Some individuals need more vitamin D than others. According to the Institute of Medicine (IOM), the safe upper limit of vitamin D is 4,000 IU per day for most adults. Check with your doctor if you think you need more vitamin D.

## Sources of Vitamin D

There are three ways to get vitamin D:

1. Supplements

2. Food

3. Sunlight

## What Is "Fortified"?

Dairy products are often labeled "fortified" with vitamin D to make them more attractive. "Fortified" means that supplements have been added to a food or beverage. Oftentimes, to reduce manufacturing costs, foods are fortified with *synthetic vitamins*.

## What Are Synthetic Vitamins?

Synthetic supplements are created in a lab to look and feel like natural vitamins and minerals, but they are anything but natural. Synthetic vitamins and minerals have negative implications on our health. Synthetic or fortified nutrients may:

- Interfere with the absorption of nutrients

**Have you ever heard that soda robs your bones?**

It is true. Most soda is high in phosphorus, a common nutrient found in our diets. In excess, phosphorus bonds with minerals like calcium, magnesium, chloride, manganese, potassium, and vitamins B and C, and zinc. Do any of these nutrients look similar to the nutrients that feed and nourish your bones?

They are. As we have learned, you need calcium, magnesium, and other essential vitamins to strengthen your bones (and muscles).

Skip the soda and feel good about preventing osteoporosis and osteoarthritis!

- Cause fat-soluble vitamins to build up in unhealthy levels

- Cause birth defects

- Cause blood clotting

- Cause hypercalcemia (buildup of calcium in the blood)

- Increase risk of cancer

Buying a generic, synthetic multi-vitamin is not going to ensure balanced calcium and vitamin D. If you think you need a supplement, first check with your doctor or a doctor who performs Nutrition Response Testing to see what you need. Then find natural supplements from a quality source rather than a synthetic variety.

## Foods Containing Vitamin D

**Sushi**–Sushi contains higher levels of vitamin D than cooked fish, but do not force yourself if you do not like raw fish; cooked varieties still offer ample amounts of the nutrient. Keep in mind that sushi rolls usually contain an overabundance of white rice, a simple carbohydrate that will fill you up without the nourishment, leading to increase in sugar cravings. When in doubt, go without (white rice, that is).

**Fish**–Canned and fresh salmon, canned and fresh mackerel, oil-packed sardines, and oil-packed tuna provide around 1/2 of the recommended daily value of vitamin D. Fish is great with vegetables, on salads, or served from the grill.

**Oysters**–Yes, I cringe at this one too, but if you like oysters, good news: Keep eating them in moderation! In addition to the 80% of your daily value in vitamin D, oysters provide a great source of copper, iron, manganese, selenium, vitamin B12, and zinc.

**Caviar** (Black and Red)–Served on whole-grain crackers or fish, caviar provides around 50% of your daily need for vitamin D per teaspoon.

**Tip from Your Trainer:** Why did I leave out soy from this list? Soy does include Vitamin D. But, soy also acts like estrogen in your body. For instance, if you have a thyroid imbalance, it may be beneficial to avoid soy products. If your soy comes from the USA, it is probably genetically modified (GMO) unless otherwise specified. Watch out for soy in things that you may not think of like chocolate, chewing gum, chips, and processed foods.

**Dairy products**–Most dairy products like milk and cheese contains small amounts of vitamin D. Always buy dairy from organic, grass-fed animals to avoid exposure to harmful chemicals. Organic diary does cost more, but you can balance the added cost by consuming *less dairy*.

**Organic eggs and mushrooms**–these foods offer a relatively low amount of vitamin D, but combined with other foods they can be an easy and delicious way to get 100% of your daily intake!

**Vitamin D supplements***–Taking a vitamin D supplement may be an important avenue if you are not getting enough of the nutrient from food or sunlight. Investigate the Consumer Reports, find a naturopath, or ask a physician (who has nutrition training) to discover which supplements are receiving high quality ratings.

*Individuals with elevated serum calcium levels or hyperparathyroidism should not take vitamin D without consulting a physician.

## Sunlight

As previously stated, your body produces vitamin D when it comes in contact with sunlight, specifically the UVB rays. Getting short, but regular exposure to sunlight can be a great (and refreshing way) to keep your bones strong and healthy. If you are concerned about skin cancer, limit your direct sun exposure and get a variety of vitamin D through food and supplementation. Talk to your physician about what the best option is for you.

## Too Much of a Good Nutrient?

As with any nutrient, stay within your recommended amounts. Too much vitamin D can put you at risk for kidney damage.

## Resistance Training for Strong Bones

What does resistance training mean to you? How is it different than cardiovascular training? Why is it relevant to weight loss and bone density?

1. According to the Harvard School of Public Health, "Strength training, also known as resistance training, weight training, or muscle-strengthening activity, *is probably the most neglected component of fitness programs but one of the most beneficial.*"

2. *Cardio training* is meant to work your *heart*, whereas *strength training* is designed to improve your *muscle tone and bone mineral density.*

### What is DOMS?

DOMS stands for delayed onset muscle soreness (post-workout muscle burn). This happens when you work out, creating surface micro-tears in your muscle. As your body repairs those tears, swelling or soreness may occur in your muscles. This is normal and usually goes away after 24-48 hours. If muscle soreness lasts for more than 3-4 days, check with your doctor to avoid injury. Reduce DOMS:

- Take an Epsom salt bath after your workout—the magnesium is beneficial for sore muscles.
- Drink the recommended amount of water per day plus an extra 20 ounces for every hour of exercise.
- Get enough vitamin C.
- Eat enough protein, complex carbohydrates, and healthy fat—especially within one hour after your workout.

## How Does Strength Training Increase Bone Mineral Density?

Bearing weight on the muscles and bones causes them to react to the stressors. The increase in your muscle seems obvious—work your muscles and they get stronger. Your bones react the same way. Put consistent, appropriate resistance on your bones and they get stronger!

Think about a tree that grows up solely in a greenhouse, sheltered from all external environments. The tree usually matures with small roots and a weak trunk. Without proper nutrients, sunshine, and natural elements such as wind and temperature, it never experiences the opportunity to fully develop. If the fragile adult tree is put outside in the wind, rain, and variable temperature, it snaps and breaks. However, if that tree is nourished and periodically taken out of the greenhouse to experience elements like wind and rain, it will grow thicker, tougher, and be able to handle its natural environment. Our bodies are similar to the trees. If we avoid resistance training and malnourish our bodies, we are at risk to bend and snap like trees grown in a greenhouse.

On the other hand, if we nourish and condition our muscles and bones to handle resistance training, they become stronger and more able to handle physical stress. Remember in Chapter 1, strength training has a multitude of benefits including:

- Reduces back pain
- Reduces stress
- Increases balance
- Improves sleep

- Reduces risk of injury
- Improves blood flow
- Improves circulation
- Improves self-image

**Tip from Your Trainer:** Muscle burns body fat. Strength training allows your body to burn fat when you are sitting at a desk, watching a movie, or even sleeping! *Strength training has benefits beyond strong bones.*

If you have not already done so, get a bone density test and a muscle percentage test (non-invasive) from a doctor and a professionally certified trainer as you start or continue strength training. Once you begin your strength routine (I hope that you have been practicing the strength workouts in this book), watch your muscle percentage and bone density increase. It is never too late to be more fit!

## No Excuses Needed

Are you stuck in a chair from bad knees? Work your upper body and core.

Are you still hurting from an old shoulder injury? Work your lower body and core.

If you can move your body, you can strengthen your body. If you do not know how to start, recruit the help of a professional.

Are you currently doing strength training?

Why or why not?

## How Much Resistance Training Should You Do Each Week?

**Trainer's Recommendation:** To improve your current physical condition, add two to three hours of strength training per week. Unless you split the workout by muscle group, the InFIT Workouts provided in this book may be performed no more than two to three times per week, as they are full body resistance training workouts (and you need at least forty-eight hours of rest between strength sessions on the same muscle groups).

If you are not currently strength training, it is not too late to start! Almost everyone can add strength training to his or her routine. The benefits far outweigh the post-exercise muscle burn.

## Practice

1. How much calcium are you consuming per day? Track for three days and record it here:

    Day 1  servings _____

    Day 2  servings _____

    Day 3  servings _____

2. How much vitamin D are you consuming per day? Track for three days and record it here:

    Day 1  IU _____

    Day 2  IU _____

    Day 3  IU _____

3. Practice adding one more day of strength training per week. What day will you exercise and which workout will you do?

_____

## S2L

Do you know a mature adult? If so, take a few moments this week to share what you learned about osteoporosis and osteoarthritis with him or her. Discuss the good news that both conditions are preventable and, in most cases, reversible! Explain the important balance of calcium and vitamin D, and how strength training builds muscle *and* bone density.

Do you follow a consistent strength training routine? _____

If so, what does it look like?

_____

If not, do you want to begin strengthening your muscles and bones?

_____

Why?

_____

What could prevent you from starting or staying consistent with your fitness goals?

_____

What can you do to overcome the Excuse Muse (Chapter 1)?

_____

Who can you review your fitness goals with?

_____

# InFIT Workout 9

First time (set) through: Warm up: Go through all of the exercises slowly, 15-20 repetitions each, with no resistance (no weight), 5-10 minutes. Second set: In the Power Level, we continue performing all three exercises in each row before moving on to the next muscle group (Lower Body, Upper Body, and Core) with minimal rest in between exercises. Perform all nine exercises and then repeat as your fitness goals and time permit! This workout incorporates a timing called TABATA. It was originally used in cardio style workouts, but TABATA is now being incorporated in strength training workouts as well. For TABATA, perform each exercise at your maximum intensity for 20 seconds and then rest for 10 seconds—repeat this eight times for each exercise. You will need a stopwatch or a clock with a second hand. Remember to stretch tight muscles before you begin.

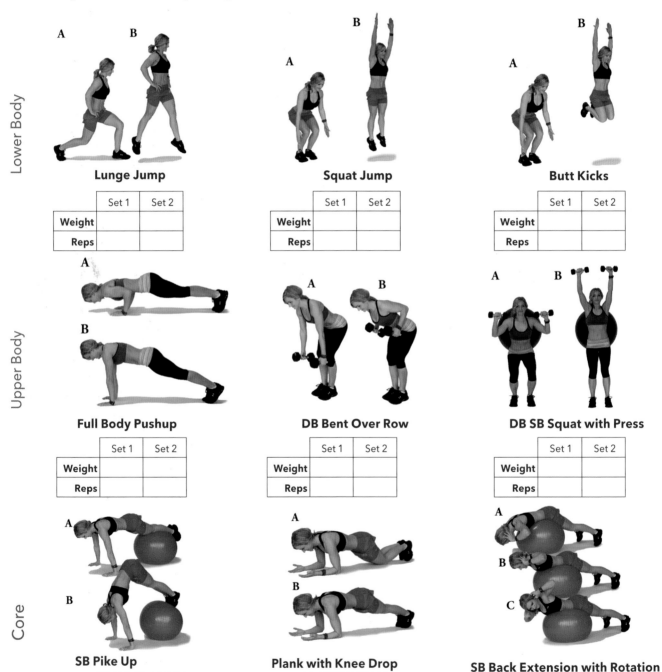

**Lower Body**

**Lunge Jump**

|  | Set 1 | Set 2 |
|---|---|---|
| Weight |  |  |
| Reps |  |  |

**Squat Jump**

|  | Set 1 | Set 2 |
|---|---|---|
| Weight |  |  |
| Reps |  |  |

**Butt Kicks**

|  | Set 1 | Set 2 |
|---|---|---|
| Weight |  |  |
| Reps |  |  |

**Upper Body**

**Full Body Pushup**

|  | Set 1 | Set 2 |
|---|---|---|
| Weight |  |  |
| Reps |  |  |

**DB Bent Over Row**

|  | Set 1 | Set 2 |
|---|---|---|
| Weight |  |  |
| Reps |  |  |

**DB SB Squat with Press**

|  | Set 1 | Set 2 |
|---|---|---|
| Weight |  |  |
| Reps |  |  |

**Core**

**SB Pike Up**

|  | Set 1 | Set 2 |
|---|---|---|
| Weight |  |  |
| Reps |  |  |

**Plank with Knee Drop**

|  | Set 1 | Set 2 |
|---|---|---|
| Weight |  |  |
| Reps |  |  |

**SB Back Extension with Rotation**

|  | Set 1 | Set 2 |
|---|---|---|
| Weight |  |  |
| Reps |  |  |

# InFIT Workout 9–Option II

During the Power level (final four workouts), we are training your reactive, fast-twitch muscle fibers, challenging your heart, and developing muscles that dynamically move in all planes of motion. In the Power Level, we continue performing all three exercises in each row before moving on to the next muscle group (Lower Body, Upper Body, and Core) with minimal rest in between exercises. *The goal is to fatigue (exhaust the muscle) after no more than 10 reps. If you can perform more than 10 reps per exercise, increase your weight.* If you find any of these exercises to be painful on your joints, please refer to a previous level's workout for safety.

**Lower Body**

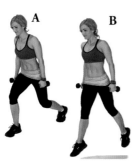

**DB Lunge Jump**

|  | Set 1 | Set 2 |
|---|---|---|
| **Weight** |  |  |
| **Reps** |  |  |

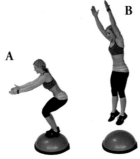

**BOSU Squat Jump**

|  | Set 1 | Set 2 |
|---|---|---|
| **Weight** |  |  |
| **Reps** |  |  |

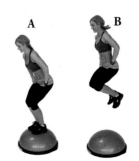

**BOSU Butt Kicks**

|  | Set 1 | Set 2 |
|---|---|---|
| **Weight** |  |  |
| **Reps** |  |  |

**Upper Body**

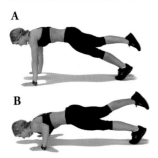

**Full Body Pushup–Single Leg**

|  | Set 1 | Set 2 |
|---|---|---|
| **Weight** |  |  |
| **Reps** |  |  |

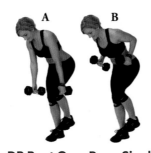

**DB Bent Over Row–Single Leg**

|  | Set 1 | Set 2 |
|---|---|---|
| **Weight** |  |  |
| **Reps** |  |  |

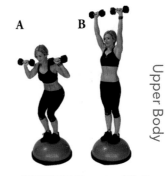

**BOSU DB Squat with Press**

|  | Set 1 | Set 2 |
|---|---|---|
| **Weight** |  |  |
| **Reps** |  |  |

**Core**

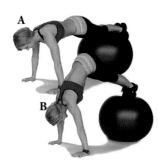

**SB Pike Up with Rotation**

|  | Set 1 | Set 2 |
|---|---|---|
| **Weight** |  |  |
| **Reps** |  |  |

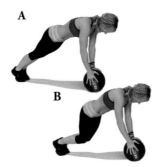

**MB Plank with Knee Drop**

|  | Set 1 | Set 2 |
|---|---|---|
| **Weight** |  |  |
| **Reps** |  |  |

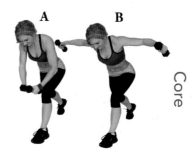

**DB Lunge with Reverse Fly**

|  | Set 1 | Set 2 |
|---|---|---|
| **Weight** |  |  |
| **Reps** |  |  |

## Review Your Map—Chapter Reflection

Use this road map as a weekly check-in to measure your goals and progress. Fill in the blank spaces at the bottom of the chart to create your own goals. The more often you check in with yourself, the more often you will bring health to the front of your mind, creating intention and success.

| GOAL | MON | TUE | WED | THU | FRI | SAT | SUN |
|---|---|---|---|---|---|---|---|
| | Actual | Actual | Actual | Actual | Actual | Actual | Actual |
| **Servings of produce (Ch 5)** | | | | | | | |
| **Water in ounces** | | | | | | | |
| **Hours of sleep (Ch 2)** | | | | | | | |
| **Minutes of exercise** | | | | | | | |
| **Weight** | | | | | | | |
| **Amount of meals/ snacks per day (Ch 3)** | | | | | | | |
| **Calories** | | | | | | | |
| **Number of simple carbs (Ch 6)** | | | | | | | |
| **Body fat % (optional)** | | | | | | | |
| **Bowel movements (Ch 8)** | | | | | | | |
| **Add your own below** | | | | | | | |
| | | | | | | | |
| | | | | | | | |
| | | | | | | | |

Did you achieve most of your goals? _____ Why? _____

What is your plan for the next week to either stay on your original course or modify based on this week's review?

How do you feel about your progress thus far?

# LIVING AFFIRMATION
## WELLNESS FOR YOUR SOUL

## The Pivotal Affirmation

Better is a dinner of herbs[a] where love is, Than a fatted calf with hatred. Proverbs 15:17

In Chapter 9 we learned about factors that are within our control and factors that are out of our control when it comes to disease. For example, we cannot control our genes or the fact that we are aging, but we can control what we eat and how much we exercise. Additionally, we cannot always control what happens to us, but we can choose the way we respond.

What are we expressing when we say we *have to* do something rather than we *choose to* do something? If people tell you how they hate it, but they *have to* work out, would you want to become their exercise buddies? How successful have you been when you told yourself that you *have to* lose weight or you *have to* eat right? Our resistant feelings set the tone for our decisions. Choosing the mindset *to want to* over *to have to* is essential in taking responsibility for our actions. At the end of the day, we are each responsible for our choices, and God is going to hold us accountable (see Genesis 3).

We can sabotage our own success with the way we approach our fitness goals. So, let's try a new approach: You *get* to work on your health. You *want* to be healthier. You *choose* to be determined. You *are* strong and able.

*How do you feel about these affirmations?*

If you agree with these affirmations, start saying them with joy!

*What new things do you want to proclaim about your life and your health?*

Be blessed abundantly! ~ *Christina Zaczkowski*, MA, CPT

## *Reflection*

_____

_____

_____

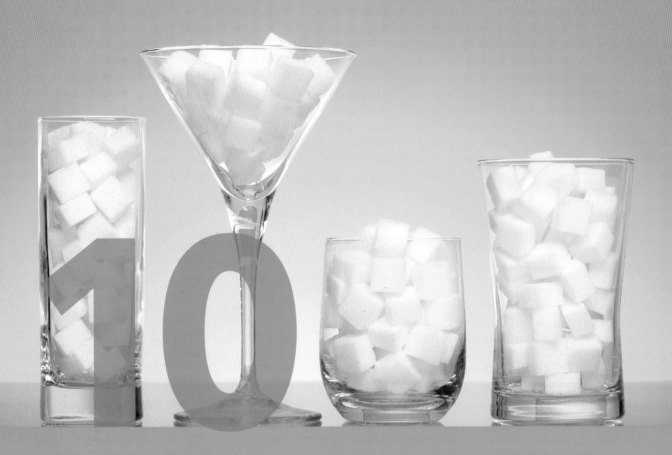

# 10

# SPORTS DRINKS, SODA & SUPPLEMENTATION, OH MY!

### Principle Questions:

1.  Is there any relationship between consuming sugar and becoming ill?

2.  Is there any harm in drinking soda or alcohol every once in a while?

3.  What are supplements? Should you take them?

4.  What supplements are right for you?

5.  How does proper supplementation help balance your nutrition?

Why did I include these topics in this book and how do they fit together? This chapter is where my story enters the stage with sugar, supplementation (or lack thereof), and illness.

I used to get sick a lot. Even as a fitness professional, my colleagues would say, "You are the healthiest sick person I know." I blamed my constant illness on bad genes and having children that brought home the bug. Sinus infections, common colds, pink-eye (yes, as an adult), strep throat, influenza, and the stomach flu. I had it all, all the time. However, there was a gradual awareness that my illnesses were wearing on my family and me. I hit the breaking point of being sick and tired over two years ago, and I have not looked back. It was in the depths of my research for this book that I decided to faithfully and consistently live out what I have been teaching for so long. When I stopped getting ill and no longer struggled with my weight, I finally understood why I was always getting sick (and battling my own weight struggles); the former me *thought* I ate enough fruits and vegetables, plenty of grains, and healthy proteins—for the most part.

*Pause.* I just said it: for the most part. Looking back during my sick and overweight years, I am honest with myself (now) that I did *not* consistently eat the enough produce, pay attention to balance healthy fats (remember the immune-boosting effects of Omega-3s and Omega-6s—see Chapter 7), drink enough water, eat all whole grains, consistently take my vitamins, learn to delegate and manage my stress, and avoid sugar like a cavity. I was a mediocre healthy person who disguised it by being *mostly* fit and *mostly* happy with my body. I had moments in my career when I hit a personal record for strength gains or even went for a month without getting a cold, but as soon as I went back to my old habits, the pounds accrued and I attracted a stomach bug.

Do you become ill more than one or two times per year?

If you become ill more than one or two times per year, take a serious look at your immune system and make changes today to improve your health.

What are some factors you attribute to your illness?

Have you ever felt sick and tired of being sick and tired?

Do you crave sugar?

Do you crave salt?

Do you think your cravings are physical, emotional, or both?

The points in this chapter have dramatically impacted my family's wellness. Life is amazing in our family when mom is healthy—everyone seems to stay healthy, and when mom is sick, everyone gets sick (leaving no one to take care of mom).

Do you feel the pain of my past illnesses? I hope not, but if you do, read on; this chapter applies to us. Imagine another scenario of sugar and malnourishment:

Your wellness and weight management program can be going great, you have figured out how many calories you need, your favorite (and least favorite) proteins, fruits, vegetables, carbs, and you have the skinny on fat (and on your skinny jeans). But then, the inevitable happens . . . you are invited and attend a party, yes, a social gathering. Perhaps you are like most people and initially uncomfortable at parties—and food and beverages are always there to comfort you. Between October and January, Americans become

## Artificial Sweeteners

Artificial sweeteners like sucralose, aspartame (NutraSweet™) and SPLENDA® cause real damage to your metabolism and your brain! Studies have shown that people who drink diet soda on a regular basis consume more calories in a day than those who drink regular soda or none at all.

Additionally, the artificial sweetener aspartame (NutraSweet™) is an excitotoxin, a chemical suggested to cause permanent damage to your brain's appetite control center.

> "I made a commitment to completely cut out drinking and anything that might hamper me from getting my mind and body together. And the floodgates of goodness have opened upon me—spiritually and financially."
>
> DENZEL WASHINGTON

extra food centric. With Halloween, Thanksgiving, Christmas, and New Year's, the food and beverages (and sugar) *add up*, while the wholesome whole foods we need are usually severely lacking—and replaced with a Russian roulette gamble with social food. We get a short break after Valentine's Day, and then we hit the Irish favorite, St. Patrick's Day, which brings us back to the topic for the chapter—sport drinks, soda pop, and supplementation (or rather the lack thereof), and other beverages at social gatherings (energy drinks and alcohol—more on alcohol in Chapter 11). Let's examine the result of drinking beverages other than water. If you are one of the healthy few who *only* drinks water, read on and help educate your friends.

## Unnecessary Calories

Do you recall in the first couple of chapters when we talked about the importance of calories? *This does not change just because it has been a few chapters.* The relationship between managing weight and managing fuel energy is still important even when you are practicing or maintaining healthy habits. In addition to unwanted calories, the sugar from sports drinks, soda, and energy drinks floods your body as highly inflammatory agents. This results in weight gain, malnourishment, and disease. What if you drink diet beverages? Does that reduce calories and sugar? One word: artificial. If your main source of sugar is artificial, you are doing your body just as much harm (or more) than if you were drinking the sugar calories. *Often we forget that beverages matter in our overall healthy lifestyle.* Ignorance is not bliss when it comes to thinking "everyone else drinks soda so it cannot be that bad, *or* the people I admire advertise it so it must not be damaging my cells." Soda and diet soda *are* that bad and everyone who drinks it is paying for the poison in their own way. Consuming excess sugar causes:

- Weight gain
- Diabetes
- Illness
- Poor nutrient absorption
- Increased triglycerides
- Heart disease
- Disease
- Depression
- Inflammation
- Poor nutrition
- Tooth decay
- Cancer

And the list goes on and on.

Go to a bookstore or Google "side effects of sugar" and read about the silent killer that few are talking about. Let's examine the details so you can make educated decisions when you pick up anything other than water to drink.

## Weight Gain. How Fast Can Calories Add Up with Light Beer?

Two 12-ounce glasses of light beer per day equals approximately:

**180** calories per day x **7** days = **1,260** extra calories per week

Three weeks equal *over 1 pound of body fat gained* from just two 12-ounce glasses of light beer a day.

When consumed, alcohol must be metabolized right away. The body will not efficiently burn sugars and fats while metabolizing alcohol. Therefore, if your beer, wine, or mixed drink is labeled 200 calories, you can be sure that the original calorie number is just a starting point (plus the extra for snacking while drinking). We will discuss more about the health risks from consuming alcohol in Chapter 11.

## Weight Gain and Soda

Two 12-ounce cans of soda per day equals approximately:

**280** calories per day x **7** days = **1,960** extra calories per week

In four weeks, over 2 pounds of body fat are *gained* from two 12-ounce cans of soda per day. Consider the reverse effect! Remove two cans of soda per day and *lose over 2 pounds of body fat in less than four weeks!* If you do not drink soda, you are not out of the fountain. Examine your diet to see if anything else might be adding extra unnecessary calories that you could reduce or remove for a significant weight loss result. Ten percent less on every plate or snack adds up to a noticeable calorie deficit quickly, allowing you to lose weight and feel satisfied without hunger pains.

## Should You Consume Sports Drinks and Energy Drinks?

Sports drinks, soda, and energy drinks are popular because of their high energy, high caffeine, and high-octane claims. However, *there is not one metabolic function in your body that requires added sugar or alcohol.* Sports drinks are meant to replace electrolytes (different kinds of sodium) during and after working out. If you work out for an hour or less, you probably do not need to replace your electrolytes *during* your workout. If you are working out for more than one hour per day (at one time), or if you are training in the heat (and you do not have time to eat a snack), you may need to balance your body's electrolytes *during* your workout. Sports drinks are a convenient way to recharge your body during or after such an endurance workout, which would be the only time I would recommend a person to consume an electrolyte drink. If you do need a beverage to fuel you, look for one with minimum sugar (5 grams or less), and no artificial colors or artificial ingredients. Remember, you are balancing your body's sodium and sugar levels, nothing more. There are many post-workout whole food options that are just as effective (if not more), and they come loaded with nutrients and fiber rather than just calories and chemicals from added sugar, color, and preservatives. Below are some of my favorite whole food combinations to replenish your body's glucose (energy), sodium chloride, and potassium after strenuous workouts—or any workout for that matter.

Do you drink energy or sports drinks?

Why?

Do you think you could replace them with any of the listed whole food options?

If so, which post-workout power foods appeal to you?

There is not one metabolic function in your body that requires added sugar.

# Post-workout Power Foods

- Ezekiel-sprouted bagel and 2 tablespoons of natural peanut or almond butter

- Celery and 2 tablespoons of natural peanut or almond butter (top with dried cherries or cranberries for an extra sweet and nutritious treat)

- Lettuce wrap with 4 ounces of chicken and 1 tablespoon of cashews (another great protein boost)

- 10 olives and 10 grapes (olives are also a great source of fiber, vitamin E, and healthy monounsaturated oils)

- Rye bread and 1 tablespoon coconut oil (Coconut oil is an anti-inflammatory—a super fuel for endurance athletes and individuals with joint pain.)

- Seaweed salad (This one may be more uncommon at home, but a great choice if you are going out to eat after your workout!)

- Sliced tomatoes, cucumbers, and real mozzarella cheese (Sodium, chloride, protein, and delicious—makes me want to go work out to enjoy this treat!)

- Banana and 2 tablespoons of natural peanut or almond butter

- Baked sweet potatoes with natural sour cream or plain Greek yogurt

- Green leafy vegetables such as spinach and kale with protein

- Homemade bean salad, avocado slices, and balsamic vinegar

These tasty meals and snacks replace your body's glucose, sodium, chloride, and potassium levels after a workout, give you *tons* of healthy protein to repair muscles, and *zero* grams of added sugar (see Chapter 6).

Now, what do sports drinks, energy drinks, alcohol, and sodas have to do with supplements? They have much in common, read on.

When we crave a food, or in this case, a beverage, it is usually a result of:

- Always eating the same foods. Lysa TerKeurst, author of *Made to Crave* says, "We crave what we eat," and it is true. If we make small changes to our nutrition, our bodies respond by craving different things. Eat a salad every day with veggies (and fruits) you like and soon you will be craving regular servings of veggies.

- Lacking an essential nutrient and looking for it from something else (like sugary beverages, alcohol, or chips).

Let's examine a few elements you may be craving and some supplements that may be able to help.

Jonny Bowden writes about the relationship between cravings and nutrient deficiencies in his book *The Most Effective Natural Cures on Earth*. Because I am not a medical doctor or nutritionist, I am not recommending any of these supplements. Check with your physician before taking supplements.

## Sugar and Glutamine

For carbohydrate, sugar, and alcohol cravings, Bowden suggests Glutamine, an amino acid that gets burned up during heavy exercise and everyday stress. Glutamine is important for immune function, intestinal health, and wound healing. A lack of glutamine can result in endurance athletes routinely getting sick after a race.

One of my colleagues braved (and finished) a 100-mile race last year. I can count on only one hand how many times he had become ill during the many years I have known him, but a day or so after his race, he was ill for a week! No doubt the lack of glutamine and other essential nutrients resulted in a real, debilitating illness. You do not have to be an ultra marathoner to experience this loss of nutrients. Exercising for two or more hours per day without resupplying your body with proper nutrition can take its toll—it has for me in the past. However when my nutrition is balanced, I do not get ill.

Glutamine can also be pivotal for those who crave alcohol. In a 1950s study on glutamine, rats who were fed glutamine consumed 35% less alcohol over the next nine days than the rats that did not consume glutamine. A 1957 study confirmed this with humans: Published in *Quarterly Journal of Studies on Alcohol*, the researchers found that 3 teaspoons of glutamine per day reduced cravings and anxiety around alcohol withdrawal by 75%.

When you have a craving for sugar or alcohol, it may be your brain craving a tangible nutrient. If you want to try glutamine, according to Bowden, take one serving under your tongue or dissolve it in a glass of water and watch the physical craving lessen.

**Tip from Your Trainer:** If plain water becomes monotonous, use the lightly flavored, tasty vitamin water recipes as alternatives to soda, sports and energy drinks, and alcohol. These water recipes are adapted from Sofia Abdelkafi.

### 1) The Classic: Lemon/Cucumber

Mix in a glass pitcher: 10 cups of water, 1 cucumber and 1 lemon, thinly sliced, and 1/4 cup fresh finely chopped basil leaves and 1/3 cup finely chopped fresh mint leaves. Leave in the refrigerator overnight before serving.

### 2) The Granite: Strawberry/Lime or Raspberry/Lime

Mix in a glass pitcher: 10 cups of water and 6 strawberries or 6 raspberries, one thinly sliced lime, and 12 finely chopped fresh mint leaves. Leave in the refrigerator overnight before serving.

> *The easiest way to be healthier (and lose weight) you will ever find is by drinking water. Sure, it sounds like you are being asked to drink a lot, but you are allowing your body to eliminate waste (fat!) and giving yourself energy. Drinking water is so simple and so important.*
>
> *When I make the effort to drink enough water daily, my body, flat out, thanks me.*
>
> MIKE S.
> REGIONAL EDITOR

**Tip from Your Trainer:**

*There are no cure-alls.* Supplement companies that suggest they have figured it all out in regards to health and fitness are lying to you and making a lot of money doing so. There are no cure-alls. A supplement that works for some may not work for everyone, as bio-individual needs vary.

My strongest recommendation is to look at what has worked for hundreds of years: whole foods, a balance of food groups, and a variety of nutrients. It is only recently that we have put our faith in processed and packaged foods and synthetic supplements and expect to live in good health.

Supplements can be a vital addition to a clean, balanced, and varied nutrition plan. But you should not use any supplements with the mind-set that they are the end-all or cure-all.

Supplements can be a great *means* to an end, but no supplement or supplement company is the end all by itself.

### 3) The Digestive: Fennel/Citrus

First: Infuse 0.1 ounce of dried and crushed fennel in 5 cups of boiling water for 5-10 minutes. Allow to cool.

Mix in a glass pitcher: 10 cups of water and lemon juice from 1 lemon (put the leftover lemon in the mix), a small thinly sliced orange, 12 fresh chopped mint leaves, and the infusion of fennel seeds. Leave in refrigerator overnight before serving.

### 4) The Antiox: Blackberry/Sage

Note that apart from the berries, sage is an herb that has the highest antioxidant content.

Mix in a glass pitcher: 10 cups of water and 1 cup of blackberries that have been slightly crushed and 3-4 sage leaves. Leave in refrigerator overnight before serving.

### 5) *Water*melon: Watermelon/Rosemary

Mix in a glass pitcher: 10 cups of water, 1 cup of watermelon cut into cubes, and 2 rosemary stems. Leave in refrigerator overnight before serving.

### 6) The Exotic: Pineapple/Mint

Mix in a pitcher: 10 cups of water, 1 cup of pineapple cut into cubes, 12 fresh mint leaves finely chopped. Leave in the refrigerator overnight before serving.

### 7) The Traditional: Apple/Cinnamon

Mix in a glass pitcher: 10 cups of water, 1 cup of apple cut into cubes, 2 cinnamon sticks, and 2 teaspoon of ground cinnamon. Leave in the refrigerator overnight before serving.

### 8.) The Zingibir: Ginger/Tea

In advance: Heat 1 teaspoon of ginger in two cups of green tea, let it cool down.

Mix in a glass pitcher: 10 cups water with the two cups of ginger infused green tea and 4-5 pieces of fresh ginger cut into cubes. Leave in the refrigerator overnight before serving.

# Magnesium

Magnesium is one of those notably necessary but often neglected nutrients in our diet. Bowden suggests magnesium as one of his "Desert Island Cures," pointing out that only three out of four Americans get the recommended daily value. Magnesium affects every cell in your body; it affects your metabolism and energy production. Not getting enough magnesium can result in any of the following problems:

- Salt and sugar cravings
- Cramps
- Insomnia
- Muscle tensions
- Poor blood sugar control
- Worsened allergy symptoms
- Cardiovascular disease
- Increased premenstrual symptoms
- Mitral valve prolapse
- Panic attacks
- Weakened immune system

This is quite a list for a rather "unknown" mineral. However, I have seen the transformation in several people, including my husband and me, with allergies, cravings, and PMS (more for me, but you know that affects him too).

Apple cider vinegar, magnesium, probiotics, fish oil (Chapter 7), and garlic are the supplements that have had the most significant impacts on my health and wellness. If I assembled a list of "Desert Island Cures," those five would be on it. However, there are no cure-alls. Apple cider vinegar, magnesium, probiotics, fish oil, and garlic positively affect my health during this season of my life. Yet, as we are all different, our bodies have different needs in regard to nutrition and supplementation. As you listen and respond to your body's needs, you will discover a balance that keeps you well. We will examine apple cider vinegar and probiotics in Chapter 11, so now let's examine garlic.

# Garlic

Allicin is the powerful antioxidant within garlic that helps maintain balanced levels of cholesterol and a healthy heart. Garlic has been used for centuries as a remedy for heart health and the treatment of common illnesses. A study dated January 2009, confirming this folk remedy in an issue of the *International Chemistry Journal Angewandte Chemie* describes garlic as one of the most powerful antioxidants available. Antioxidants are responsible for fighting free radicals, reversing signs of aging, and killing bacteria in your body. Add a clove to your veggies, salad, or chicken breast to fight toxic-free radicals in your body instantly. The less you cook garlic, the higher the antioxidant value will be. However, if you do not love the flavor of fresh garlic, try lightly steaming it with your veggies to begin to train your pallet!

# Why Is Sodium Important?

As we discussed earlier in this chapter, sodium plays an important role in the regulation of your body's electrical and nerve functions. Sodium also plays a vital role in regulating nutrients in and out of every cell in your body and regulating your blood pressure. Because of the real buzz words "heart disease," we as a nation are afraid of salt. Many people avoid sodium because of the link to heart disease. The problem is not sodium. The problem is either *too much* sodium from processed foods or not enough sodium because we are afraid of it.

Are you still drinking enough water per day (half of your ideal body weight in ounces)?

If not, what prevents you from drinking enough water?

What are the *essential* benefits from drinking the proper amount of water?

What are the real consequences of *not* drinking enough water?

Tip from Your Trainer: If plain water becomes monotonous, use this chapter's tasty treats separate or together to add some flavor and spice to your water:

- Basil
- Cucumber slices
- Lemon juice
- Lime juice
- Orange slices
- Apple cider vinegar

When we do not get enough sodium, the result is hyponatremia, which is a metabolic condition where the salt and water is dangerously out of balance between the inside and outside of our cells.

One of my colleagues recently passed out at my fitness center. His trauma is one of the scariest things I have been through. He was teaching a class when he felt off balance. He went to the bathroom to try to regain control of his shaky body and he fainted. We called for an ambulance as he remained unconscious. He was brought to the hospital for a battery of tests for his heart, lungs, and brain. After checking all his body's vitals, blood counts, and minerals, he was diagnosed with hyponatremia. Hyponatremia can be life threatening and may cause:

- Brain herniation
- Death
- Possible coma

I do not point this out to scare you. I shared this real event so that, similar to my colleague, so you can take great care in getting *enough* and the *right kind* of salt in your diet.

## Sodium in Packaged Foods versus Added Mineral Salt

Two ways to ingest sodium are from:

1. Processed and packaged foods
2. Adding salt to your home-cooked foods

*I strongly encourage you to avoid processed and packaged foods.*

You should run from sodium in packaged foods because of all the other poisonous chemicals that accompany most convenience foods. Most Americans eat packaged and processed foods as though they are candy so we do not usually worry about *low* sodium. However, because I am encouraging you to *avoid* packaged and processed foods and make choices that involve more whole foods, *this choice must come with an understanding that sodium is an essential mineral*. Be sure to salt your meals with quality mineral salt to get the appropriate amount of salt your body needs.

## How Much Sodium Do We Need?

"The *2010 Dietary Guidelines for Americans* recommends limiting sodium to less than 2,300 milligrams a day—or 1,500 milligrams if you are age 51 or older, if you are black, or if you have high blood pressure, diabetes, or chronic kidney disease, according to the Mayo Clinic. Track your sodium for up to three days to find out how much you are consuming; it may surprise you. Getting enough, but not overdoing sodium is an essential part of feeling good, protecting your heart, and stepping off of the "sick and tired" roller coaster.

## What Are Good Sources of Sodium?

- Salt

- Cheese

- Saltwater crab

- Homemade soup

- Celtic sea salt (especially for low thyroid functioning conditions)

- Pink Himalayan salt (Think: Most of the time, real salt has a color!)

If you think you are low in any of the above supplements, check with your doctor to see if adding one or more may be beneficial to help manage your weight, help manage your cravings, and help get you off the roller coaster of "sick and tired."

## Iodine in Salt

Iodine is an essential nutrient for your body. Iodine is marketed on some table salt as a great "source" of the nutrient. However, the iodine found in most table salt (sodium chloride) is synthetic and although we might be fooled, our bodies are not. Consuming synthetic iodine usually results in an iodine deficiency and a potentially under-functioning thyroid *due to* a constant exposure to elements that cause an imbalance in your body's essential nutrients. Most manufacturers are looking for the cheapest way to mass-produce foods and condiments we use every day. Instead of obtaining iodine through fortified salt, iodine should be consumed naturally from foods like sea salt, kale, egg yoke, tuna, garlic, asparagus, and spinach to name a few. Rather than choosing table salt, go to the source—mineral salt. It is nourishing and gives your body the balance of minerals it is looking for.

## Balanced Body. Balanced Mind.

If there were no connection to what we put in our bodies and how we felt, the supplementation industry would crash. The fact is, *what* we put into our bodies *does* impact how we feel. Let me repeat that, *what we put into our bodies impacts how we feel*.

Supplementation is a billion-dollar industry because most people want to live longer and feel better. We want to lose weight and look younger. My best advice for your bio-individual supplementation is to find a holistic nutritionist, a doctor who offers Nutrition Response Testing, or a naturopath who is recommended and trusted. Get tested to find out specifically what your body needs during various seasons, what

**Notes**

nutrients it absorbs well, and what it does not. Until you receive an individual supplementation plan, make sure your body's most essential nutrients are balanced. Remember, health is a way of life, not a temporary or fad diet.

## Practice

1. If you are drinking anything with added sugar, reduce your consumption by half for three days and then get rid of it altogether for three days and document how you feel—you may feel challenged by withdrawal the first few days, so stick with it and watch your energy and immune system soar.

How did you feel when you reduced your sugar intake by half?

_____

_____

How did you feel when you avoided added sugar in drinks for three days?

_____

_____

2. What is one benefit of magnesium?

_____

_____

3. How much sodium do you need per day?

_____

_____

## S2L

Acknowledge your food or beverage cravings (if any) and discuss them with a friend. Based on what you know, offer a few explanations to your cravings. Explain the danger of consuming too much sugar and not enough sodium. Encourage them to achieve balance in their nutrition by eating the recommended servings of produce, carbohydrates, protein, and fat, and by limiting PPC: processed, packaged, and convenience foods whenever possible.

Track your milligrams (mg) of sodium for three days and record it here:

Day 1  mg _____

Day 2  mg _____

Day 3  mg _____

Discuss strategies to balance your sodium intake.

**Notes**

# InFIT Workout 10

First time (set) through: Warm up: Go through all of the exercises slowly, 15-20 repetitions each, with no resistance (no weight), 5-10 minutes. Second set: In the Power Level, we continue performing all three exercises in each row before moving on to the next muscle group (Lower Body, Upper Body, and Core) with minimal rest in between exercises. Perform all nine exercises and then repeat as your fitness goals and time permit! For workout 10, we focus on power and proprioception. (Remember the benefits of balance include brain health and injury prevention.) This time, however, the moves are more challenging. If you find any of these exercises to be painful on your joints, please refer to a previous level's workout for safety. Remember to drink water during your workout and stretch tight muscles.

## Lower Body

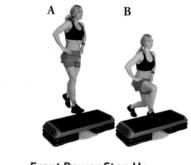

**Front Power Step Up**

|  | Set 1 | Set 2 |
|---|---|---|
| Weight |  |  |
| Reps |  |  |

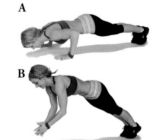

**Speed Jump Squat**

|  | Set 1 | Set 2 |
|---|---|---|
| Weight |  |  |
| Reps |  |  |

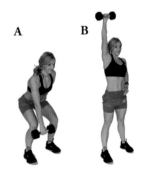

**DB Snatch**

|  | Set 1 | Set 2 |
|---|---|---|
| Weight |  |  |
| Reps |  |  |

## Upper Body

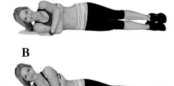

**Single Arm Side Push Up**

|  | Set 1 | Set 2 |
|---|---|---|
| Weight |  |  |
| Reps |  |  |

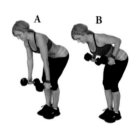

**Plyometric Push Up**

|  | Set 1 | Set 2 |
|---|---|---|
| Weight |  |  |
| Reps |  |  |

**DB Speed Bent Over Row**

|  | Set 1 | Set 2 |
|---|---|---|
| Weight |  |  |
| Reps |  |  |

## Core

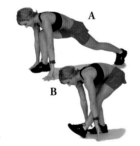

**Speed Runner's Start to Lunge**

|  | Set 1 | Set 2 |
|---|---|---|
| Weight |  |  |
| Reps |  |  |

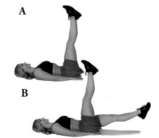

**Speed Scissor**

|  | Set 1 | Set 2 |
|---|---|---|
| Weight |  |  |
| Reps |  |  |

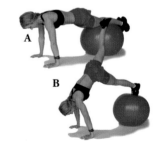

**SB Single Leg Pike Up**

|  | Set 1 | Set 2 |
|---|---|---|
| Weight |  |  |
| Reps |  |  |

# InFIT Workout 10—Option II

In the Power Level, we continue performing all three exercises in each row before moving on to the next muscle group (Lower Body, Upper Body, and Core) with minimal rest in between exercises. Perform all nine exercises and then repeat as your fitness goals and time permit!

Lower Body

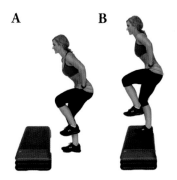

**Front Power Jump Up to Balance**

|  | Set 1 | Set 2 |
|---|---|---|
| Weight |  |  |
| Reps |  |  |

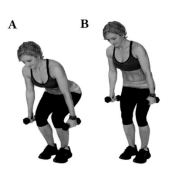

**DB Speed Squat**

|  | Set 1 | Set 2 |
|---|---|---|
| Weight |  |  |
| Reps |  |  |

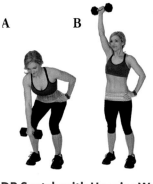

**DB Snatch with Heavier Weight**

|  | Set 1 | Set 2 |
|---|---|---|
| Weight |  |  |
| Reps |  |  |

Upper Body

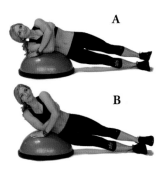

**BOSU Single Arm Side Push Up**

|  | Set 1 | Set 2 |
|---|---|---|
| Weight |  |  |
| Reps |  |  |

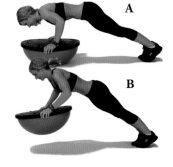

**BOSU Plyometric Push Up**

|  | Set 1 | Set 2 |
|---|---|---|
| Weight |  |  |
| Reps |  |  |

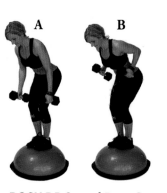

**BOSU DB Speed Bent Over Row**

|  | Set 1 | Set 2 |
|---|---|---|
| Weight |  |  |
| Reps |  |  |

Core

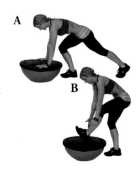

**BOSU Speed Runner's Start to Lunge**

|  | Set 1 | Set 2 |
|---|---|---|
| Weight |  |  |
| Reps |  |  |

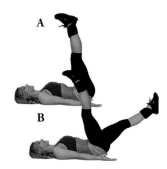

**Speed Scissor with Ankle Weights**

|  | Set 1 | Set 2 |
|---|---|---|
| Weight |  |  |
| Reps |  |  |

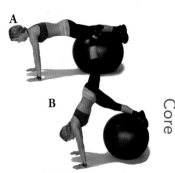

**SB Single Leg Pike Up with Ankle Weights**

|  | Set 1 | Set 2 |
|---|---|---|
| Weight |  |  |
| Reps |  |  |

# ROAD MAP TO **SUCCESS**

## Review Your Map—Chapter Reflection

Use this road map as a weekly check-in to measure your goals and progress. Fill in the blank spaces at the bottom of the chart to create your own goals. The more often you check in with yourself, the more often you will bring health to the front of your mind, creating intention and success.

| | GOAL | MON | TUE | WED | THU | FRI | SAT | SUN |
|---|---|---|---|---|---|---|---|---|
| | | Actual | Actual | Actual | Actual | Actual | Actual | Actual |
| **Servings of produce (Ch 5)** | | | | | | | | |
| **Water in ounces** | | | | | | | | |
| **Hours of sleep (Ch 2)** | | | | | | | | |
| **Minutes of exercise** | | | | | | | | |
| **Weight** | | | | | | | | |
| **Amount of meals/ snacks per day (Ch 3)** | | | | | | | | |
| **Calories** | | | | | | | | |
| **Number of simple carbs (Ch 6)** | | | | | | | | |
| **Body fat % (optional)** | | | | | | | | |
| **Bowel movements (Ch 8)** | | | | | | | | |
| **Add your own below** | | | | | | | | |
| | | | | | | | | |
| | | | | | | | | |
| | | | | | | | | |

Did you achieve most of your goals? _____ Why? _____

What is your plan for the next week to either stay on your original course or modify based on this week's review?

How do you feel about your progress thus far?

# LIVING AFFIRMATION
WELLNESS FOR YOUR SOUL

## Our Job

Naked I came from my mother's womb, and naked shall I return there. The Lord gave, and the Lord has taken away; Blessed be the name of the Lord. Job 1:21

Perhaps you have heard the Old Testament story about Job, who was righteous in the sight of God and led a good life. On the day he learned that his children were killed and his livestock stolen, he did not curse God—he reminded his soul that God is the giver of everything and people should not think that they own anything before God. Later, however, on the day that Job lost his good health, there was no stopping him from cursing the day he was born. What a sad twist to the story! Alone, losing his kids, his wife, and his livestock did not shake Job's faith, but combined with losing his health to painful sores all over his body, Job hated his very existence. In the end, God showed himself to Job and answered all Job's questions with the revelation of God's authority over everything. Job's story makes me wonder what it takes for a person to be shaken to the core and make changes in life. It is gripping to me that Job needed to become sick in order to be shaken to the core.

For Job to have questioned the God he served all his life, his health had to have been severely compromised. *What happened in your life to make you question the status of your health?*

It is our job to be honest with God and ourselves. We want to be healthy. Please take time and reflect on what it took for you to realize it was time to change the state of your health. If you are not yet intentionally traveling toward a healthy lifestyle, maybe you would benefit from thinking about what it would take for you to get there. You may be surprised what you find out about yourself.

Be blessed abundantly! ~ *Christina Zaczkowski*, MA, CPT

## *Reflection*

_____

_____

_____

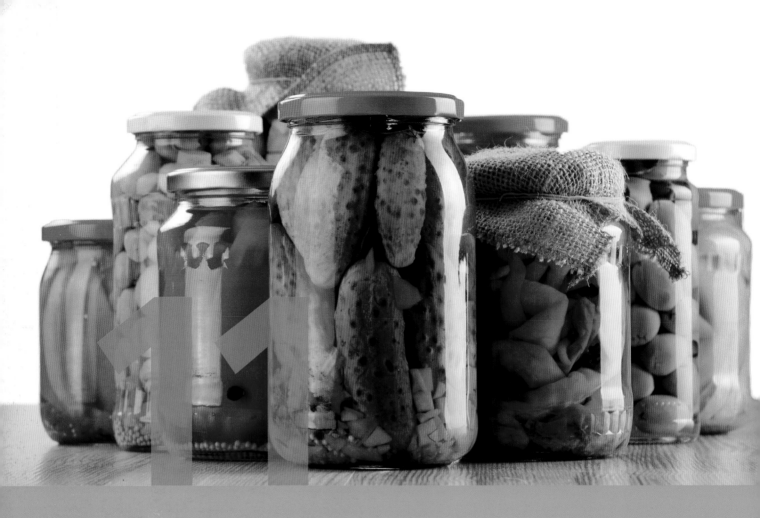

# FERMENTATION
## Living Foods for Better Digestion
## Watch Your Foods Come to Life!

### Principle Questions:

1.  How long have we been fermenting food and beverages? What is fermentation?

2.  What are examples of fermented foods and beverages?

3.  What are the benefits of fermentation?

4.  What are the dangers of not consuming fermented foods or beverages?

5.  How do you make fermented foods?

Fermentation has been around since ancient times and has been studied extensively since the 1500s with the invention of the compound microscope. Fermentation is the process of adding microorganisms such as mold, yeast, or bacteria to foods and beverages to break down or digest compounds and nutrients. Your body does this naturally when you eat food; your stomach naturally produces chemicals to break down your food. Yet, often we do not have enough natural bacteria (flora) in our stomach or some foods (grains and proteins) need more assistance than others to break down and digest. Fermented foods and beverages are an integral part of proper digestion.

Examples of fermented foods and beverages include:

- Cider and vinegar

- Yogurt, kefir, and some cultured cheese

- Certain breads like sourdough and ciabatta

- Pickled vegetables (Examples: sauerkraut, pickles, beets, et cetera)

- Wine, beer, and other alcoholic beverages

*A trainer once said in a session,"You will be amazed what you can train your body to do!" The impact of those few words has lasted and will carry me forever.*

JONE B.
ANYTIME FITNESS H2I

## Benefits of Pre-digested Foods and Beverages (Fermentation)

Fermented foods help your body break down and absorb nutrients, boost your immune system, and keep your bowels regular. Fermented foods also support necessary bacteria in our digestive tract. Your body's natural supply of flora gets crushed from certain medications, chlorinated water, and antibiotics in our foods; we need good bacteria on a daily basis to keep the balance of flora in our bodies.

Remember when we compared our metabolism to a flow of traffic in Chapter 2? Think of that flow of traffic again and imagine if the cars traveling through the streets and intersections were the food in our bodies, and the necessary bacteria are the stoplights. If you do not have any stoplights (lack of bacteria from consuming too much chlorine in tap water or antibiotics in meat and dairy), the streets would get congested and backed up with cars (constipation). When there are too many cars in one place for too long, chemicals like carbon dioxide start to build up (*bad* bacteria in our stomachs). Car jams and congested roads lead to polluted cities and frustrated people. When we cannot digest our food, the same toxicity and constipation occurs in our bodies.

For example, imagine eating a few slices of pizza knowing they will sit and rot in your gut for a couple of days if they do not digest properly. They become like magnets for disease-causing bacteria. Where are the stoplights to keep that pizza flowing through your body in a timely manner? A healthy portion of fiber will help move the pizza along, but *not until the pizza is broken down* will it travel all the way through the digestive tract. Healthy bacteria and fermented foods and beverages will help to digest the pizza so that the fiber you ate can take the garbage out to the trash.

If you have ever heard that a 6-ounce glass of wine per day is good for you, the benefits of fermentation support that statement. But, as in all good things, *more than what is beneficial* means harmful. Limit your consumption of alcoholic beverages and instead focus on consuming a *variety* of fermented foods and beverages. If you do not drink alcohol, there is no need to start. Too much alcohol adds calories and a host of other negative side effects, including nerve damage, liver damage, heart damage, brain damage, withdrawal, damage to unborn children, and sexual disorders. There are many other ways to incorporate fermented foods into your nutrition plan:

- Add organic vinegar to your salad or steamed veggies.

- Occasionally replace your regular bread with a fresh sourdough variety.

- Add kefir or yogurt to your smoothies.

- Try drinking Kombucha—a fermented beverage found in grocery and whole food stores.

- Add fermented vegetables like pickled cucumbers, beets, kimchi, onions, salsa, and sauerkraut to meals and snacks.

- Add a tablespoon of fermented chutney to cooked poultry or beef.

- Try fermenting your own foods! Have the courage to discover what you like and what you do not.

## Homemade Sauerkraut

The following is Sandor Ellix Katz easy sauerkraut recipe from his book *Wild Fermentation: The Flavor, Nutrition, and Craft of Live-Culture Foods* (Chelsea Green, 2003).

Timeframe: One to four weeks (or more)

### Special Equipment

Ceramic crock or food-grade plastic bucket, 1 gallon capacity or greater

Plate that fits inside crock or bucket

1-gallon jug filled with water (or a scrubbed and boiled rock for weight)

Cloth cover (like a pillowcase or towel)

*"Fortune favors the bold."*

ALEXANDER THE GREAT

### Ingredients (for 1-gallon jug)

5 pounds cabbage

3 tablespoons sea salt

### Process

Chop or grate cabbage, finely or coarsely, with or without hearts, however you like it. I love to mix green and red cabbage to end up with bright pink kraut. Place cabbage in a large bowl as you chop it.

Sprinkle salt on the cabbage as you go. The salt pulls water out of the cabbage (through osmosis) and this creates the brine in which the cabbage can ferment and sour without rotting. The salt also has the effect of keeping the cabbage crunchy, by inhibiting organisms and enzymes that soften it. Three tablespoons of salt is a rough guideline for five pounds of cabbage. I do not measure an exact amount of salt; I shake it on after I chop up each cabbage. I use more salt in summer, less in the winter.

Add other vegetables. Grate carrots for a coleslaw-like kraut. Other vegetables I include are onions, garlic, seaweed, greens, Brussels sprouts, small whole heads of cabbage, turnips, beets, and burdock roots. You can also add fruits (apples, whole or sliced, are classic) and herbs and spices (caraway seeds, dill seeds, celery seeds, and juniper berries are delicious, but anything you delight in will work). Experiment!

Mix ingredients together and pack into a crock. Pack just a bit into the crock at a time and tamp it down hard using your hands or a sturdy kitchen utensil. The tamping packs the kraut tight in the crock and helps force water out of the cabbage.

Then, cover kraut with a plate or some other lid that fits snugly inside the crock. Place a clean weight (a glass jug filled with water) on the cover. This weight is to force water out of the cabbage and then keep the cabbage submerged under the brine. Cover the whole thing with a cloth to keep debris out.

Press down on the weight to add pressure to the cabbage and help force water out. Continue this periodically (as often as you think of it, every few hours), until the brine rises above the cover. This can take up to twenty-four hours, as the salt draws water out of the cabbage slowly. Some cabbage, particularly if it is old, simply contains less water. If the brine does not rise above the plate level by the next day, add enough salt water to bring the brine level above the plate. Add about a teaspoon of salt to a cup of water and stir until it is completely dissolved.

Leave the crock to ferment. I generally store the crock in an unobtrusive corner of the kitchen where I will not forget about it, but where it will not be in anyone's way. You could also store it in a cool basement if you want a slower fermentation that will preserve longer.

Check the kraut every day or two. The volume reduces as the fermentation proceeds. Sometimes mold appears on the surface. Many books refer to this mold as "scum," but I prefer to think of it as a bloom. Skim what you can off of the surface; it will break up and you will probably not be able to remove all of it. Do not worry about this. It is just a surface phenomenon, a result of contact with the air. The kraut itself is under the anaerobic protection of the brine. Rinse off the plate and the weight. Taste the kraut. In the cool temperatures of a cellar in winter, kraut can keep improving for months and months. In the summer or in a heated room, its life cycle is more rapid. Eventually it becomes soft and the flavor turns less pleasant. Generally it starts to be tangy after a few days, and the taste gets stronger.

I generally scoop out a bowl or jar full at a time and keep it in the fridge. I start when the kraut is young and enjoy its evolving flavor over the course of a few weeks. Try the sauerkraut juice that will be left in the bowl after the kraut is eaten. Sauerkraut juice is a rare delicacy and unparalleled digestive tonic. Each time you scoop some kraut out of the crock, you have to repack the kraut carefully. Make sure the kraut is packed tight in the crock, the surface is level, and the cover and weight are clean. Sometimes brine evaporates, so if the kraut is not submerged below the brine, just add salted water as necessary. Some people preserve kraut by canning and heat-processing it. Heat kills the healthy, living properties of the kraut: Avoid heat when you can.

Develop a rhythm. I try to start a new batch before the previous batch runs out. I remove the remaining kraut from the crock, repack it with fresh salted cabbage, then pour the old kraut and its juices over the new kraut. This gives the new batch a boost with an active culture starter.

Enjoy!

Tip from Your Trainer: Avoid eating three hours before bed—especially foods with sugar, natural or added. Eating an apple right before bed can cause the sugars in the apple to ferment in your stomach, leading to dangerous health risks, including cancer.

## Practice

Your goal should be to maintain your body's flora through whole foods and beverages. If you think you need a probiotic, check with your physician. It is possible to get too much good bacteria in your stomach. If you experience bloating, gas, and diarrhea, you may have had too much sauerkraut, alcohol, or vinegar. Listen to the signs and symptoms of your body and take control of your health.

1. How does your gut feel today?

_____

Have you had any fermented foods lately?

_____

2. Try three new fermented foods this week and document how you feel.

_____

## S2L

Discuss the benefits of fermented foods with a friend. Who will you share your thoughts with and what will you discuss?

_____

List three examples of fermented foods.

_____

_____

_____

# Christina's Famous "Sauerkraut Auflauf" Story and Recipe

In the past, I did not like sauerkraut—I know, that is un-German of me. Leaving Germany, learning more about optimal nutrition, missing my mother's comforting cuisine, and being asked all the time if I eat sauerkraut, I found myself trying to reconstruct my mother's famous sauerkraut dish.

It turns out to be prepared almost in a dash of salt (I love that in a recipe!) and Americans love this dish where ever I have served it!

All you need is some red-skinned potatoes (lower starch levels), organic butter, sauerkraut (you will find the balance you like if you make it a couple of times. I would go for less grams of potatoes than sauerkraut), a fresh pineapple or canned in its own juice, and shredded cheese (I prefer pepper jack).

## Action Plan:

- Boil (to peel or not to peel, that is your preference!) potatoes until soft to make mashed potatoes with an appropriate amount of organic butter.

- While the potatoes boil, drain one serving of sauerkraut.

- Cut up pineapple or open can and drain the juice (or drink the juice).

- Cut up bits of meat or decide to serve meat on the side.

- Start preheating oven to 425 degrees Fahrenheit.

- When potatoes are mashed, spread flat on the bottom of a deep-dish pan.

- Spread pineapple chunks over the mashed potatoes.

- Spread the sauerkraut next.

- Finish with shredded cheese on top.

- Put into oven until cheese is golden to brown (about 15-20 minutes).

You can barely mess this dish up—it is so simple. I hope you will enjoy it! The sauerkraut will beautifully help your gut digest what has already been through your digestive system that day. Guten Appetit! (German for "Enjoy your meal!")

Original recipe from Christina Zaczkowski

# InFIT Workout 11

First time (set) through: Warm up: Go through all of the exercises slowly, 15-20 repetitions each, with no resistance (no weight), 5-10 minutes. Second set: In the Power Level, we continue performing all three exercises in each row before moving on to the next muscle group (Lower Body, Upper Body, and Core) with minimal rest in between exercises. Perform all nine exercises and then repeat as your fitness goals and time permit! Plyometric training (jump training) continues in workout 11 for cardio and strength integration. If you find any of these exercises to be painful on your joints, please refer to a previous level's workout for safety. Remember to drink water during your workout and stretch tight muscles.

## Lower Body

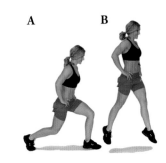

**Lunge Jump ALT Legs**

|        | Set 1 | Set 2 |
|--------|-------|-------|
| Weight |       |       |
| Reps   |       |       |

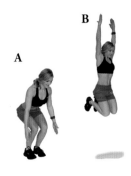

**Butt Kicks**

|        | Set 1 | Set 2 |
|--------|-------|-------|
| Weight |       |       |
| Reps   |       |       |

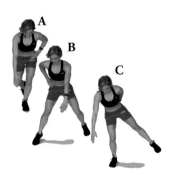

**Ice Skater**

|        | Set 1 | Set 2 |
|--------|-------|-------|
| Weight |       |       |
| Reps   |       |       |

## Upper Body

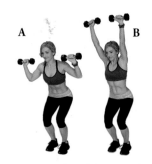

**DB ISO Squat with Speed Press**

|        | Set 1 | Set 2 |
|--------|-------|-------|
| Weight |       |       |
| Reps   |       |       |

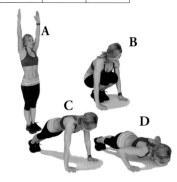

**Burpees with Pushup**

|        | Set 1 | Set 2 |
|--------|-------|-------|
| Weight |       |       |
| Reps   |       |       |

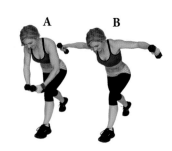

**DB ISO Lunge with Speed Reverse Fly**

|        | Set 1 | Set 2 |
|--------|-------|-------|
| Weight |       |       |
| Reps   |       |       |

## Core

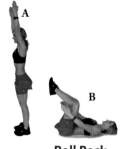

**Roll Back**

|        | Set 1 | Set 2 |
|--------|-------|-------|
| Weight |       |       |
| Reps   |       |       |

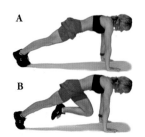

**Mountain Climber**

|        | Set 1 | Set 2 |
|--------|-------|-------|
| Weight |       |       |
| Reps   |       |       |

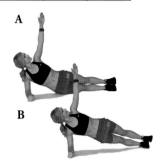

**Speed Full Side Plank**

|        | Set 1 | Set 2 |
|--------|-------|-------|
| Weight |       |       |
| Reps   |       |       |

# InFIT Workout 11—Option II

In the Power Level, we continue performing all three exercises in each row before moving on to the next muscle group (Lower Body, Upper Body, and Core) with minimal rest in between exercises. Perform all nine exercises and then repeat as your fitness goals and time permit!

**Lower Body**

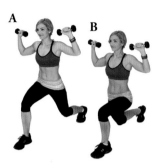

### Lunge Jump ALT Legs with DB Shoulder Press

|        | Set 1 | Set 2 |
|--------|-------|-------|
| Weight |       |       |
| Reps   |       |       |

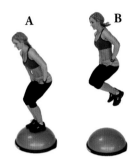

### BOSU Butt Kicks

|        | Set 1 | Set 2 |
|--------|-------|-------|
| Weight |       |       |
| Reps   |       |       |

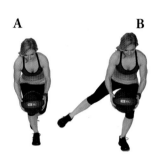

### MB Ice Skater

|        | Set 1 | Set 2 |
|--------|-------|-------|
| Weight |       |       |
| Reps   |       |       |

**Upper Body**

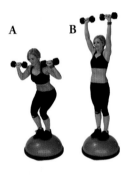

### BOSU DB Squat with Speed Press

|        | Set 1 | Set 2 |
|--------|-------|-------|
| Weight |       |       |
| Reps   |       |       |

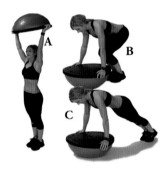

### BOSU Burpees with Pushup

|        | Set 1 | Set 2 |
|--------|-------|-------|
| Weight |       |       |
| Reps   |       |       |

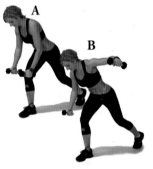

### DB ISO Lunge with Speed Reverse Fly–Single Arm

|        | Set 1 | Set 2 |
|--------|-------|-------|
| Weight |       |       |
| Reps   |       |       |

**Core**

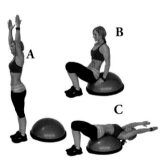

### BOSU Roll Back

|        | Set 1 | Set 2 |
|--------|-------|-------|
| Weight |       |       |
| Reps   |       |       |

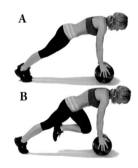

### MB Mountain Climber

|        | Set 1 | Set 2 |
|--------|-------|-------|
| Weight |       |       |
| Reps   |       |       |

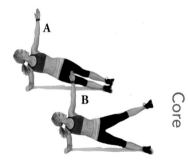

### Speed Full Side Plank with Leg Extension

|        | Set 1 | Set 2 |
|--------|-------|-------|
| Weight |       |       |
| Reps   |       |       |

# ROAD MAP TO **SUCCESS**

## Review Your Map–Chapter Reflection

Use this road map as a weekly check-in to measure your goals and progress. Fill in the blank spaces at the bottom of the chart to create your own goals. The more often you check in with yourself, the more often you will bring health to the front of your mind, creating intention and success.

| | GOAL | MON Actual | TUE Actual | WED Actual | THU Actual | FRI Actual | SAT Actual | SUN Actual |
|---|---|---|---|---|---|---|---|---|
| Servings of produce (Ch 5) | | | | | | | | |
| Water in ounces | | | | | | | | |
| Hours of sleep (Ch 2) | | | | | | | | |
| Minutes of exercise | | | | | | | | |
| Weight | | | | | | | | |
| Amount of meals/ snacks per day (Ch 3) | | | | | | | | |
| Calories | | | | | | | | |
| Number of simple carbs (Ch 6) | | | | | | | | |
| Body fat % (optional) | | | | | | | | |
| Bowel movements (Ch 8) | | | | | | | | |
| **Add your own below** | | | | | | | | |
| | | | | | | | | |
| | | | | | | | | |
| | | | | | | | | |

Did you achieve most of your goals? _____ Why? _____

What is your plan for the next week to either stay on your original course or modify based on this week's review?

How do you feel about your progress thus far?

# LIVING AFFIRMATION
## WELLNESS FOR YOUR SOUL

## Filing Chapter 11

Owe no one anything except to love one another, for he who loves another has fulfilled the law.
Romans 13:8

Legally, filing Chapter 11 is a form of bankruptcy that involves admitting the need for assistance in dealing with debt. It can also offer a fresh start to rebuild over the course of time. Bankruptcy and rebuilding is not achieved without transparency.

Bankruptcy affects one of the most intimate aspects of our lives: our freedom, our families, and our resources. In the same way fermentation affects one of the most intimate parts of our body: the gut; our digestion, our absorption, and elimination. Fermented foods offer assistance to our digestive system when we do not treat our gut as it requires to be healthy.

*Have you been transparent, or do you need to file Chapter 11 with God?*

Filing bankruptcy with God means admitting our shortcomings and giving God permission to reorganize the business of our life so that God's name will be glorified.

Be blessed abundantly! ~ *Christina Zaczkowski*, MA, CPT

## *Reflection*

_____

_____

_____

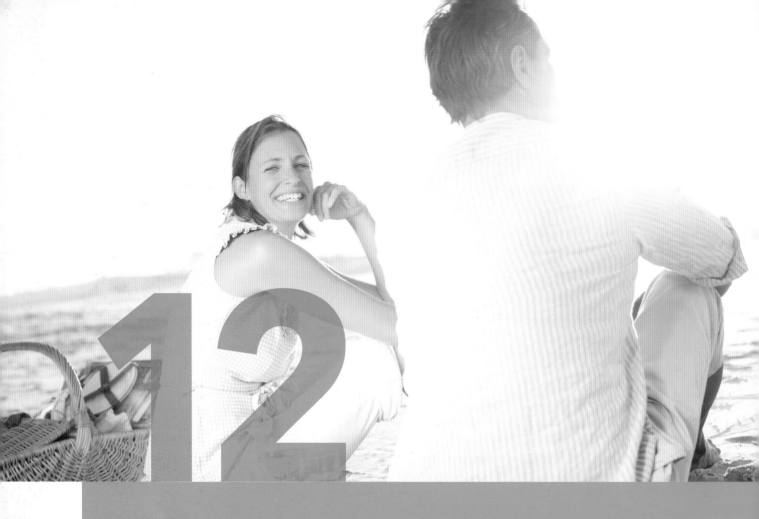

# 12

# A WHOLE, HEALTHY YOU
## From the Inside Out!

### Principle Questions:

1.  What is your Big Picture for health?

2.  Why is it crucial to review your past goals?

3.  What have you learned? How have you grown (or shrunk)?

4.  What are your new short-term goals? What are your new long-term goals?

5.  Do you believe you are worth optimal health?

You made it through the whole book! (Or maybe you just flipped to the final chapter to see how it felt to make it through the whole book.) Wherever you are in your journey, congratulate yourself that you are, or have been practicing, becoming a more healthy, happy you, from the inside out.

When looking back at the Big Picture, healthy food and beverages, protein and carbohydrates, supplements and fermentation, it may feel as though they all do the same things—health is simple right? Not exactly: An important concept from this book is that each element we have examined has a *unique* and *essential* function.

For example, fruits and vegetables nourish your cells; fermented foods help break down the nutrients and absorb them; protein rebuilds cells after they have been damaged; fat and carbohydrates fuel your muscles and brain; fiber collects toxins and waste from your body and ushers it out through the intestines; and supplementation fills in the gaps of vitamins and minerals your body may not be receiving or absorbing through food. Each puzzle piece of health plays its part, and they all work together to create a whole, healthy you—from the inside out. Instead of following the temptation of the Excuse Muse or allowing the fear that optimum health is too hard to maintain, believe and trust that you were created for more, that you can learn new healthy habits as you did when you were a child, and continue becoming the healthiest you that you can be.

I titled this chapter "A Whole, Healthy You From the Inside Out" because you have journeyed long and far to get here, and you have another exciting choice ahead of you.

My hope and prayer for you is that you have seen the fruit of your labor over the past several weeks or months, that you will continue on the journey toward optimal health, and that you will share the secrets you have learned with others. Let's reflect on the journey we have taken together and assess your current situation before we move forward with a new, exciting plan.

## Reviewing the Plan

As you review your original plan, have any of your goals changed? Often when I begin a journey, I have a vision of what I *hope* and *think* is going to happen along the way. However, with health and fitness, I notice that my goals usually *change* the more I learn. As I learn more about myself, I discover who I want to become, often resulting in a positive deviation from my original plan.

Have you changed course along the way? Yes/No

Why?

My hope and prayer for you is that you have seen the fruit of your labor over the past several weeks or months, that you will continue on the journey toward optimal health, and that you will share the secrets you have learned with others.

Our journey toward health and wellness began with a nutrition and fitness assessment. Mark this page and flip back to Chapter 1 to review your past thoughts, mindsets, and goals.

What were your short-term (one to six months) nutrition goals?

1. _____

2. _____

3. _____

*One year ago, my goal was to lose wight. Yet, after reading* Living Wellness, *weight loss was no longer my main goal.*

*Learning about nutrition and fitness helped me realize my new goal of becoming the healthiest person I can be. Now I desire to eat right and understand what my body needs to function my best every day.*

*I enjoy teaching my children and my family everything I learn so they can make choices to be healthy and have Living Wellness become a part of their lifestyle.*

CARMEN T.
INFIT DIRECTOR

*And you shall know the truth, and the truth shall make you free.*

JOHN 8:32

Have you moved toward these goals in a healthy, productive way?

_____

What were your long-term (six months to one year) nutrition goals?

1. _____
2. _____
3. _____

## Physical Fitness

What were your short-term (zero to six months) fitness goals?

1. _____
2. _____
3. _____

What were your long-term (six months to one year) fitness goals?

1. _____
2. _____
3. _____

Have you moved toward these goals in a healthy, productive way? How?

_____

How do you feel about yourself and your journey (think about your mind, body, and soul)?

_____

_____

What have you learned over the course of this book? Flip back through the previous chapters to read your notes.

_____

_____

What habits and mindsets have you changed?

_____

_____

What habits and mindsets do you still struggle with?

_____

_____

Are you a healthier person now than when you started your journey?

_____

Change takes time. You may not even be six months into your transformation. Think back to when you (or someone you know) learned how to ride a bicycle. How can you forget, right? If you were like me, it was hard work, painful, and often frustrating, especially if you had an older sibling who was beyond your skills and enjoyed pointing out your shortcomings in learning.

Once you practiced and became comfortable on the bike, you could take one hand off the bike, one foot off the bike, close your eyes for a moment or two, and then eventually you just felt *free*. Free to ride without a care in the world, free to know you were confident on the bike when you steered, when you turned, and when you rode over an unexpected bump. I remember the feeling of freedom so clearly since that moment. The pain and work of learning how to ride my bike paid off. Have I fallen off and gotten hurt since? Yes. If I could go back, I would do it all over again for the exhilarating freedom of riding my bike. The falls become less frequent with time and practice and enjoyment of the activity grows. I loved (and still love) riding my bike, but there was a lot of hard work and discipline to enjoy the freedom I have now.

Our health journey is similar to learning how to ride a bike. In the beginning there is uncertainty, doubt, pain, struggle, time, and perceived failure, but eventually, there is knowledge. Knowledge offers choices and making consistent, sound decisions develops discipline. There is freedom in discipline. I am not talking about a strict set of rules or a "do this" and "do not do that" approach to health and wellness. I am talking about a lifestyle. I was purposeful to use language like "try this" and "avoid that." *Food is not evil. Discipline is not a dirty word.*

The more we learn and practice disciplining our bodies, minds, and attitudes, the stronger they become and the more freedom we gain. I want to be free. Do you want to be free?

Do you want to count calories every day for the rest of your life? *No, probably not.*

Do you want to look at every food label for the rest of your life? *No, that is too time consuming.*

Do you want to avoid restaurants forever because you cannot handle temptations and the thought of making terrible choices scare you? *No, I hope not.*

My prayer and desire is that *Living Wellness* guides you in this phase of your health journey and that it enables you to confidently make statements like: *I know my body's needs, the signs of hunger*

## Positive Self-Talk

Practicing your part in health includes knowing the importance of positive self-talk:

Positive self-talk is a crucial part of endurance in your wellness journey. You have an *opportunity* to be healthier; it is not a chore or a curse. You have the *ability* to make choices; you are not hopeless in your current situation. You have the *strength* to honor your body with physical activity, rather than dreading another workout. Repeat these phrases:

- I *get to* be healthier.
- I make wise choices.
- I am strong and I enjoy moving my body in the way it was designed.
- I am created for more than mediocre health.
- Or, make up your own!

Practice daily, positive self-talk until it becomes habit and reality.

*and thirst, and the nutrients I need to be balanced from the inside out. I confidently walk through the grocery store with freedom, plan my meals with ease, and eat out with friends and family when I want. I choose to exercise because I am worth optimal fitness.* This is freedom. It comes with practice and discipline. Agreeing with God that your health is important and freely becoming a good steward of your body allows health to become a joyful journey.

Alongside freedom comes the reward of health. Were any of your goals to feel better, look better, have more energy, have less pain, sleep better, have less disease, be more confident, and achieve and maintain a healthy weight?

Did you begin to grasp those goals? Have you made a breakthrough yet? Are you more healthy now than when you started? Did you set out on your trip with appropriate goals, adequate support, and a backup plan for setbacks? If you did, you are now eating better, moving more, feeling better, and you have likely improved your physical health and your weight. If you are not there yet, *do not panic*. Do not even feel disappointed! Guilt has no place here. Keep moving forward.

Think about the child learning to ride a bicycle as if it were your child. What if they practiced for days and weeks and still could not figure out how to ride? What would you tell the child? *I guess riding a bike is just not for you. Try again when you are less busy. I guess you were just born that way, time to accept it.* No! You would encourage, offer suggestions, say *practice again*, believe in, help and guide, and then celebrate in his or her success. You are somewhere on that bicycle! Now is not the time to stop riding. It is not time to put the road map down. Keep practicing your part in health to receive a breakthrough no matter where you are in your journey.

The following excerpt is from Mark Batterson's book *The Circle Maker* on the challenge of breakthrough:

"I had the privilege of hearing Chuck Yeager recount his experiences at the Smithsonian National Air and Space Museum with Parker's Cub Scout Troop. Right outside the IMAX Theater where Yeager gave the speech, the Bell X-1 is symbolically suspended in midair, along with other historic aircraft and spacecraft. Each one represents a breakthrough. Each one is a testament to the ingenuity and irrepressibility of the human spirit, which of course, is a gift of the Holy Spirit.

Just like the sound barrier, there is a faith barrier. And breaking the faith barrier in the spiritual realm is much like breaking the sound barrier in the physical realm. If you want to experience a supernatural breakthrough, it often feels like you're about to lose control, about to fall apart. That is when you need to press in and pray through. If you allow them to, your disappointments will create drag. If you allow them to, your doubts will nosedive your dreams. But if you pray through, God will come through and you'll experience supernatural breakthrough."

This parallel of breaking through a sound barrier and a spiritual barrier is a powerful illustration. Think about those astronauts preparing to launch into space. There is fear, excitement, anticipation, and thoughts of the unknown. Once the 1,607,185 pounds of solid rocket boosters were ignited, there was an unbelievable amount of noise, pressure, and trembling. Imagine yourself in the launch seat! Have you allowed the challenge and the pressure of your health efforts to prevail? Did you offer your fear up to God and have faith that there will be a breakthrough? If so, wow, what a journey! Breakthroughs are scary, but they bring freedom and reward. Breakthroughs bring an ease and comfort knowing you worked hard, you had faith, and *achieved something worthwhile*. With God's help, anything is possible. If you are feeling the pressure of the engines and the awareness of uncertainty, *press in, pray, and have faith*. A breakthrough is up ahead.

## Practice—Looking Ahead

What are your *new* short-term (one to six months) health goals?

_____

_____

_____

_____

What are your *new* long-term (six months to one year) health goals?

_____

_____

_____

_____

How have you started overcoming the Excuse Muse?

_____

_____

**Enjoying Freedom**

What will you do (or have you been doing) with your newfound energy and vitality? (Examples: start dancing, volunteer, join a recreational athletic team, play with your children, run with your dog, et cetera).

*Exercise and fitness help channel my excess energy from negative to positive. They keep me balanced and out of trouble!*

Dawn V.
InFIT instructor

*For God has not given us a spirit of fear, but of power and of love and of a sound mind.*

2 Timothy 1:7

*I will praise You, for I am fearfully and wonderfully made.*

Psalm 139:14

*Let us accept the gift of our bodies and be excited for our amazing journey ahead.*

**Notes**

Who have you discussed your goals with in the past?

_____

_____

_____

Will you continue sharing your goals with them in the future? Yes/No

Do you believe you can become even healthier?

_____

_____

_____

Why?

_____

_____

_____

*Do you believe you are worth the challenge of breaking through tough habits, perhaps even life-long habits, for better health?*

Review this book often. The more you bring health front of mind, the more your wellness becomes a top priority. You now know what to do to be a healthier person. Practicing consistent healthy habits makes for a lifetime of improvement. Think how often parents must remind children to brush their teeth when they are young! After 999,999 times, I think my children finally understand the importance and they do it without thinking (although very occasionally they still need reminding). *We too, need reminding.* We need to hold one another accountable and hold one another up to a standard above average, because right now, there is nothing healthy about average.

*Do you believe you are worth exceptional health of your mind, body, and soul?*

You *are* worth it. I know you are worth it. You deserve exceptional health and wellness. "For God has not given us a spirit of fear, but of power and of love and of a sound mind." 2 Timothy 1:7. This verse is for you. It means that you have been given all the tools necessary to be healthy, including common sense (a sound mind)! "I will praise You, for I am fearfully and wonderfully made." Psalm 139:14. You are the most beautiful creation God has ever made. Let us accept the gift of our bodies and be excited for the amazing journey ahead.

May God richly bless you on your continued journey.

*Ashley R. Darkwhite*

Notes

# InFIT Workout 12

First time (set) through: Warm up: Go through all of the exercises slowly, 15-20 repetitions each, with no resistance (no weight), 5-10 minutes. Second set: In the Power Level, we continue performing all three exercises in each row before moving on to the next muscle group (Lower Body, Upper Body, and Core) with minimal rest in between exercises. Perform all nine exercises and then repeat as your fitness goals and time permit! Our final InFIT Workout incorporates stabilization, strength, power, and balance. If you find any of these exercises to be painful on your joints, please refer to a previous level's workout for safety. Remember to drink water during your workout and stretch tight muscles.

## Lower Body

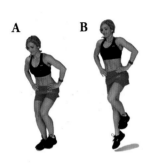

### Lunge Jump–Single Leg

|  | Set 1 | Set 2 |
|---|---|---|
| Weight |  |  |
| Reps |  |  |

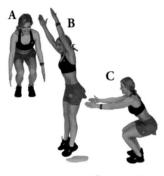

### Jump Squat with Rotation

|  | Set 1 | Set 2 |
|---|---|---|
| Weight |  |  |
| Reps |  |  |

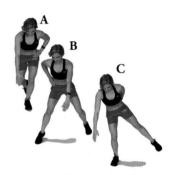

### Speed Ice Skater to Balance

|  | Set 1 | Set 2 |
|---|---|---|
| Weight |  |  |
| Reps |  |  |

## Upper Body

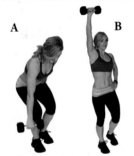

### DB Snatch–Single Leg

|  | Set 1 | Set 2 |
|---|---|---|
| Weight |  |  |
| Reps |  |  |

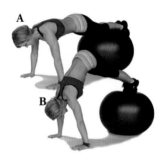

### SB Speed Pike Up

|  | Set 1 | Set 2 |
|---|---|---|
| Weight |  |  |
| Reps |  |  |

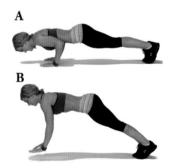

### Plyometric Triceps Pushup

|  | Set 1 | Set 2 |
|---|---|---|
| Weight |  |  |
| Reps |  |  |

## Core

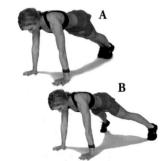

### Speed Plyometric Prone Jack

|  | Set 1 | Set 2 |
|---|---|---|
| Weight |  |  |
| Reps |  |  |

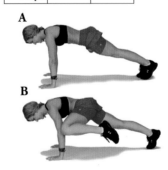

### ISO Plank Military Pushup

|  | Set 1 | Set 2 |
|---|---|---|
| Weight |  |  |
| Reps |  |  |

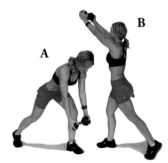

### DB Chop and Lift

|  | Set 1 | Set 2 |
|---|---|---|
| Weight |  |  |
| Reps |  |  |

# InFIT Workout 12–Option II

In the Strength Level, we continue performing all three exercises in each row before moving on to the next muscle group (Lower Body, Upper Body, and Core) with minimal rest in between exercises. Perform all nine exercises and then repeat as your fitness goals and time permit!

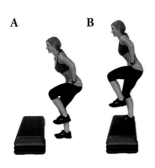

**Single Leg Jump Up to Step**

|        | Set 1 | Set 2 |
|--------|-------|-------|
| Weight |       |       |
| Reps   |       |       |

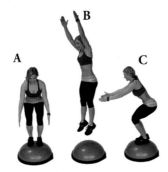

**BOSU Jump Squat with Rotation**

|        | Set 1 | Set 2 |
|--------|-------|-------|
| Weight |       |       |
| Reps   |       |       |

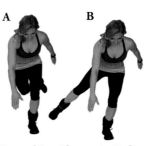

**Speed Ice Skater to Balance with Ankle Weights**

|        | Set 1 | Set 2 |
|--------|-------|-------|
| Weight |       |       |
| Reps   |       |       |

Lower Body

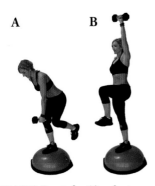

**BOSU DB Snatch–Single Leg**

|        | Set 1 | Set 2 |
|--------|-------|-------|
| Weight |       |       |
| Reps   |       |       |

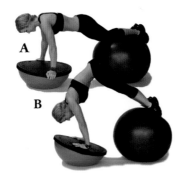

**BOSU SB Speed Pike Up**

|        | Set 1 | Set 2 |
|--------|-------|-------|
| Weight |       |       |
| Reps   |       |       |

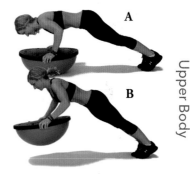

**BOSU Plyometric Triceps Pushup**

|        | Set 1 | Set 2 |
|--------|-------|-------|
| Weight |       |       |
| Reps   |       |       |

Upper Body

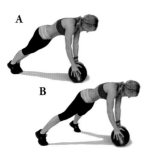

**MB Speed Plyometric Prone Jack**

|        | Set 1 | Set 2 |
|--------|-------|-------|
| Weight |       |       |
| Reps   |       |       |

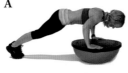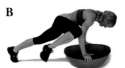

**BOSU ISO Plank Military Pushup**

|        | Set 1 | Set 2 |
|--------|-------|-------|
| Weight |       |       |
| Reps   |       |       |

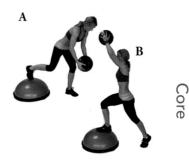

**BOSU MB Chop and Lift**

|        | Set 1 | Set 2 |
|--------|-------|-------|
| Weight |       |       |
| Reps   |       |       |

Core

## Review Your Map—Chapter Reflection

Use this road map as a weekly check-in to measure your goals and progress. Fill in the blank spaces at the bottom of the chart to create your own goals. The more often you check in with yourself, the more often you will bring health to the front of your mind, creating intention and success.

| | GOAL | MON Actual | TUE Actual | WED Actual | THU Actual | FRI Actual | SAT Actual | SUN Actual |
|---|---|---|---|---|---|---|---|---|
| **Servings of produce (Ch 5)** | | | | | | | | |
| **Water in ounces** | | | | | | | | |
| **Hours of sleep (Ch 2)** | | | | | | | | |
| **Minutes of exercise** | | | | | | | | |
| **Weight** | | | | | | | | |
| **Amount of meals/ snacks per day (Ch 3)** | | | | | | | | |
| **Calories** | | | | | | | | |
| **Number of simple carbs (Ch 6)** | | | | | | | | |
| **Body fat % (optional)** | | | | | | | | |
| **Bowel movements (Ch 8)** | | | | | | | | |
| **Add your own below** | | | | | | | | |
| | | | | | | | | |
| | | | | | | | | |
| | | | | | | | | |

Did you achieve most of your goals? _____ Why? _____

What is your plan for the next week to either stay on your original course or modify based on this week's review?

How do you feel about your progress thus far?

# LIVING AFFIRMATION
## WELLNESS FOR YOUR SOUL

## A Memorable Good-Bye

Being confident of this, that he who began a good work in you will carry it on to completion until the day of Christ Jesus. Philippians 1:6

If you had one last piece of wisdom to pass on to someone, what would you say? Here are my parting words to you: *God does not give up on people.*

God does not give up on you, nor anyone you would call a hopeless case. God desires for everyone to know His love! When we give God permission, God changes our lives. We are granted forgiveness from our mistakes and the consequences of our mistakes. He wants to bring our relationships into order, heal our hearts, and transform our minds.

He has great plans for you. In God, we find our specific purpose and have abundant and eternal life. We are all works in progress. God is good, and you can trust Him.

I pray that the Holy Spirit reveals Jesus Christ to you in new ways, to the joy of our Father! I pray that you would not settle for anything less than an abundant quality of life (as Jesus promised in John 10:10). And I pray that your eyes and heart be opened to the expectation of your best physical and spiritual health.

Be blessed abundantly! ~ *Christina Zaczkowski*, MA, CPT

## *Reflection*

_____

_____

_____

# WISDOM FROM THE PAGES

- People by and large become what they think about themselves. Bob Rotella

- To be physically healthy, people will realize that they must take care of their inner being. To be healthy within, people will realize that they must take care of their physical body. Harold Eberle

- *You are the only one who can make the decision to become the person you were designed to be.*

- *If you know how much energy your body needs, you will be able to make wiser choices.*

- *I have never met one person who is 100% happy with his or her body. Let us love and honor our bodies the way they are right now and watch our exteriors transform out of love, rather than self-hatred.*

- *No one has perfect eating habits. Let's not make that our goal. Let us make our goal to eat cleaner and healthier than we did yesterday.*

- The saddest thing, I think, amongst all common but tragic ironies, is to feel fat and very hungry at the same time. Unknown

- *Look for food that will nourish you, not just provide fuel.*

- *While it may look good on the surface to sacrifice yourself, you are not doing anyone a favor, including yourself. When our health suffers, when our depression rises and our bodies fail us, who can we help? Who can we serve when we have no more energy? If we neglect our responsibility for our health, the cost will probably be paid by the next generation.*

- *Optimal nutrition is not about, "is this food good or bad." Optimal health is about choosing your best option in the given circumstance.*

- By failing to prepare, you are preparing to fail. Benjamin Franklin

- *Out of sight . . . Keep junk food out of the house! "Out of sight, out of mind" is an effective motto.*

- *If ice cream is your weakness, do not buy ice cream. If you eat a whole bag of chips in one sitting, avoid buying chips until you have established discipline—or do not buy them at all. Save yourself money and buy a good pair of running shoes instead.*

- Just because you do not have much to choose from, does not mean you cannot choose wisely. Jay Shearer

- *When grocery shopping, remember to get a variety of fresh, frozen, canned, and dried or dehydrated produce and meat so you can stay focused when you run out of fresh, whole foods.*

- *Weight Management Benefits: Protein satisfies, keeps you full longer, and uses more energy to digest than other fuel sources.*

- Do not let your fire go out, spark by irreplaceable spark in the hopeless swamps of the not-quite, the not-yet, and the not-at-all. Do not let the hero in your soul perish in lonely frustration for the life you deserved and have never been able to reach. The world you desire can be won. It exists . . . it is real . . . it is possible . . . it's yours. Ayn Rand

- *Remember, protein rebuilds and repairs all cells, not just muscle cells.*

- *Most healthy recipes take less time to prepare than waiting for pizza delivery.*

- *Notice how you can eat certain packaged foods like ice cream and chips until the package is empty? When was the last time you finished the entire bag of lettuce or polished off three apples? If you keep craving a certain food after one serving, it may be time to pick a different food. Produce is satisfying.*

- But until a person can say deeply and honestly, "I am what I am today because of the choices I made yesterday," that person cannot say, "I choose otherwise." Stephen R. Covey

- *The cost savings from eating clean are real. They are not just "pie in the sky" suggestions that may or may not happen with improved health. When you fuel and nourish your body with the right foods and the right amounts, you will be healthier. You will feel better. You will save money, short-term and long-term.*

- We were made to crave—long for, want greatly, desire eagerly, and beg for—God. Only God. Lysa TerKeurst, *Made to Crave*

- It's not the "how to" I'm missing. It's the "want to". . . really wanting to make changes and deciding that the results of those changes are worth the sacrifice. Lysa TerKeurst

- *The less added sugars and simple carbs you consume, the less your body will crave them AND you will have the added benefit of your body using fat as a main fuel source, rather than mostly sugar (glucose).*

- *The more sugar we eat, the more we crave.*

- *Like anything worthwhile, we need time and discipline to practice making better choices, but they get easier, and there is little more important and permanent than the health of you and your children's brains.*

- *Remember, food is energy. If it does not get used, it gets stored!*

- Medical failings: Medical doctors, to whom we have entrusted out health because we have not yet learned to care for it ourselves, studied disease rather than health in medical school. Their curriculum included little on nutrition, lots on pharmaceutical drugs, and nothing about the effects of processing fats and oils on human health. Udo Erasmus

- *Hence, we need more Omega-3s and less Omega-6s in our diets until we have cleaned up and kicked out the majority of packaged foods in our pantries.*

- *The fat from healthy oils like fish and walnuts hold oxygen in our cells. Certain viruses, bacteria, fungi, and other foreign organisms cannot live in the presence of oxygen. Optimal intakes of healthy fat has a very tangible, positive effect on our immune system.*

- *If we consumed the recommended amount of fruits, veggies, and water per day, the fiber supplement industry would crash overnight.*

- The opposite of love is not hate, it's indifference. The opposite of beauty is not ugliness, it's indifference. The opposite of faith is not heresy, it's indifference. And the opposite of life is not death, but indifference between life and death. Elie Wiesel

- A merry heart does good, like medicine,[a] But a broken spirit dries the bones. Proverbs 17:22

- Let food be thy medicine and medicine be thy food. Hippocrates

- *Let us see the scale for what it is: a measure of how much you weigh, not a measure of your worth.*

- I made a commitment to completely cut out drinking and anything that might hamper me from getting my mind and body together. And the floodgates of goodness have opened upon me-spiritually and financially. Denzel Washington

- *Not one metabolic function in your body requires added sugar.*

- *Supplements can be a great means to an end, but no supplement or supplement company is the end all by themselves.*

- *What we put into our bodies impacts how we feel.*

- Fortune favors the bold. Alexander the Great

- *Changing your pallet opens you to new flavors, textures, and spices.*

- *My hope and prayer for you is that you have seen the fruit of your hard work over the past several weeks or months, that you will continue on the journey toward optimal health, and that you will share the secrets you have learned with others.*

- And you shall know the truth, and the truth shall make you free. John 8:32

- For God has not given us a spirit of fear, but of power and of love and of a sound mind. 2 Timothy 1:7

- I will praise you, for I am fearfully and wonderfully made. Psalm 139:14

- *Let us accept the gift of our bodies and be excited for our amazing journey ahead.*

- Being confident of this very thing, that He who has begun a good work in you will complete it until the day of Jesus Christ. Philippians 1:6

# GROCERY LIST FOR MEAL PLANNING

Beverages – herbal tea, water, sparkling water, 100% fruit juice, et cetera

- 
- 
- 
- 

Bread/Bakery – 100% whole-grain items (sprouted when available)

- 
- 
- 
- 

Canned/Jarred Goods – vegetables, spaghetti sauce, fruit, almond butter, ketchup (avoid additives)

- 
- 
- 
- 

Dairy – butter, cheeses, eggs, milk, yogurt (from organic, grass-fed animals when available)

- 
- 
- 
- 

Dry/Baking Goods – rice, beans, nuts

- 
- 
- 
- 

Frozen Foods – meat, vegetables, fruit

- 
- 
- 
- 

Meat – fish, poultry, beef, pork (avoid preservatives)

- 
- 
- 
- 

Produce – fruits, vegetables (organic when available)

- 
- 
- 
-

Household Products (What you use in use in home and on your body is important–choose the most natural household products available)

- 
- 
- 
- 

Cleaners – all-purpose laundry detergent, dish washing liquid/detergent (look for brands like Norwex with no fillers)

- 
- 
- 
- 

Paper Goods – paper towels, toilet paper, aluminum foil, sandwich bags

- 
- 
- 
- 

Personal Care – shampoo, soap, hand soap, shaving cream (avoid carcinogens like ethanolamines and parabens)

- 
- 
- 
- 

Other – baby items, pet items, batteries, greeting cards, et cetera

- 
- 
- 
- 
- 
- 
- 
- 
- 
- 
- 
- 
- 
- 
- 
- 
- 
- 
- 
- 
-

# MEAL PLANNING IN CIRCLES!

Use the circles below to plan your meals for one week. You do not always need one food in every food group for every meal and snack, but give it a try and see how it goes!

## Breakfast

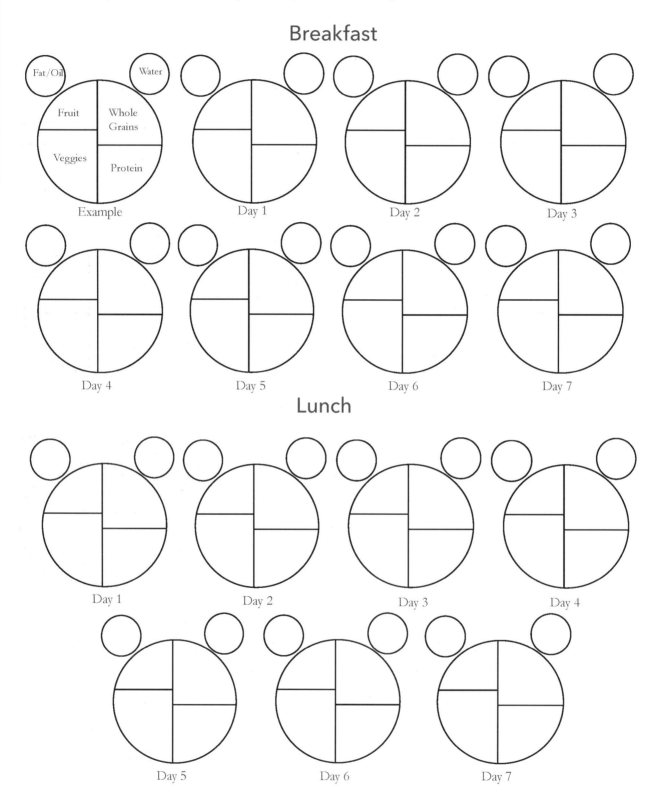

Fat/Oil    Water

Fruit    Whole Grains

Veggies    Protein

Example    Day 1    Day 2    Day 3

Day 4    Day 5    Day 6    Day 7

## Lunch

Day 1    Day 2    Day 3    Day 4

Day 5    Day 6    Day 7

# Dinner

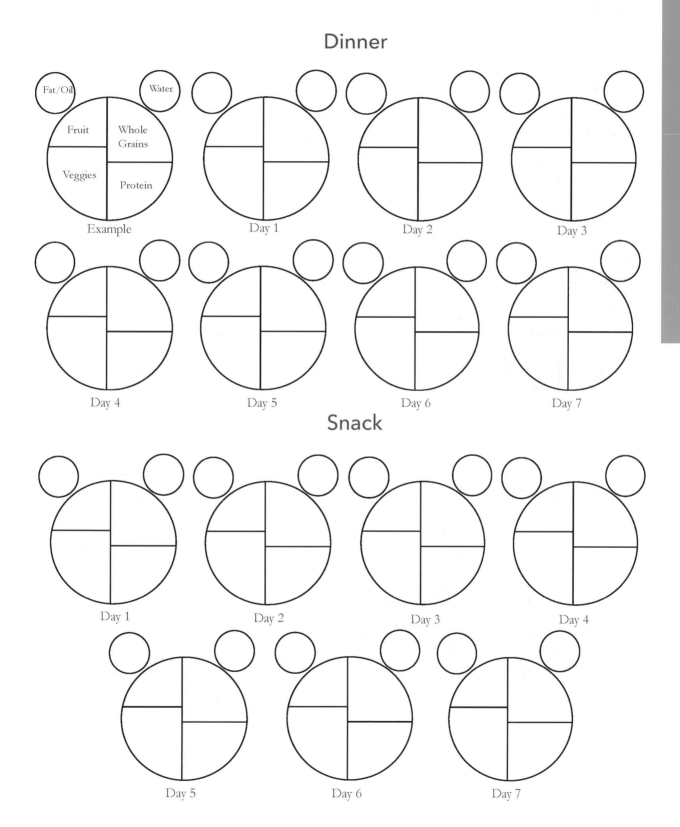

Fat/Oil | Water

Fruit | Whole Grains

Veggies | Protein

Example | Day 1 | Day 2 | Day 3

Day 4 | Day 5 | Day 6 | Day 7

# Snack

Day 1 | Day 2 | Day 3 | Day 4

Day 5 | Day 6 | Day 7

# EXPANDED INGREDIENTS TO AVOID

## Added Sugar

Corn syrup and high fructose corn syrup

Dextrose

Fructose

Galactose

Maltose

Sucrose

White sugar

## Artificial Colors

## Artificial Preservatives

BHA and BHT

Nitrates and nitrites

Partially hydrogenated oil

Potassium bromate

Sodium benzoate

Sodium nitrate and sodium nitrite

Sulfates and sulfites

## Enriched/Refined Grains

## Flavor Enhancers

Artificial Sweeteners

Aspartame

Monosodium Glutamate (MSG)

Sodium cyclamate

SPLENDA®

Sucralose

## Stick Margarine

## Shortening

# PERCEIVED RATE OF EXERTION CHART

## Instructions for Borg Rating of Perceived Exertion (RPE) Scale

While doing physical activity, we want you to rate your perception of your exertion. This feeling should reflect how heavy and strenuous the exercise feels to you, combining all sensations and feelings of physical stress, effort, and fatigue. Do not concern yourself with any one factor such as leg pain or shortness of breath, but try to focus on your total feeling of exertion.

Look at the rating scale below while you are engaging in an activity; the scale ranges from 6 to 20, where 6 means "no exertion at all" and 20 means "maximal exertion." Choose the number from below that best describes your level of exertion. This will give you a good idea of the intensity level of your activity, and you can use this information to speed up or slow down your movements to reach your desired range. If you are not wearing a heart rate monitor, this scale is useful to determine if you are practicing cardiovascular exercise or physical activity (see Chapter 1). Cardiovascular exercise occurs approximately at an exertion of 13 or more.

Try to appraise your feeling of exertion as honestly as possible without thinking about what the actual physical load is. Your own feeling of effort and exertion is important, not how it compares to others. Look at the scale and the expression and then give a number.

**9** corresponds to "very light" exercise. For a healthy person, it is comparable to walking slowly at his or her own pace for some minutes.

**13** on the scale is "somewhat hard" exercise, but it still feels ok to continue.

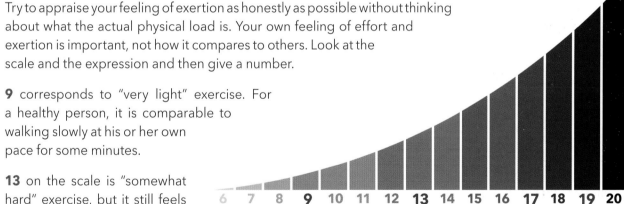

6  7  8  **9**  10  11  12  **13**  14  15  16  **17**  18  **19**  **20**

NO EXERTION AT ALL                                   MAXIMAL EXERTION

**17** "very hard" is very strenuous. A healthy person can still go on, but he or she really has to push him- or herself. It feels very heavy, and the person is very tired. Examples of this exertion are kettlebells, trail racing, or intense rowing.

**19** on the scale is an extremely strenuous exercise level. For most people this is the most strenuous exercise they have ever experienced. Labor and delivery, or sprinting for extended periods of time are examples of this level of exertion.

Borg RPE scale © Gunnar Borg, 1970, 1985, 1994, 1998

# PRACTICE SECTIONS, CHAPTER BY CHAPTER

## Chapter 1

1. Keep a wellness journal. Make it personal by writing important objectives for your health, nutrition, exercise, sleep, body composition, feelings, successes, challenges, et cetera. If you track your nutrition electronically, I encourage you to keep a separate wellness journal on a computer or notebook. Take this opportunity to get to know yourself and your body.

2. Make a plan. How often are you going to work out?

_____

_____

What time of day are you going to work out?

_____

_____

3. What is your backup plan if that time of day does not fit?

_____

_____

## Chapter 2

1. Continue recognizing why you eat. Are you hungry? Are you thirsty? Are you bored? Are you addicted? Are you sad? Is your body lacking a nutrient? Is food available in the staff room at work or on the kitchen counter? When you recognize the signals of your body, you are able to make better choices. Consistently healthy choices lead to better health (and usually weight loss if that is one of your goals).

2. Ninety-five percent of your food should be for nourishment. Treats should be saved for rare and special occasions. Before you reach for your next meal or snack, ask yourself, will this food or beverage nourish my body or is it simply providing fuel or pleasure?

3. Read labels. If you do not have time to read every single label (I recommend eventually getting in this habit) at the store, start by reading all of your breakfast labels and avoid added sugar, artificial colors, flavors, and preservatives. Look for whole grains and whole foods for breakfast instead of colorful, sugary cereal (remember that study on artificial colors and children). Your family may not be happy with your nutritional changes, but consider that any change is challenging at first. I promise the payoff is worth the practice.

# Chapter 3

1.  Track your progress. Continue tracking your calories and choose food for fuel and nourishment.

2.  Build variety. When grocery shopping, pick up a variety of fresh, frozen, canned, and dried produce and protein to avoid turning to junk food when you run out of fresh, whole foods or for convenience.

3.  Think ahead. Plan out your meals a couple of days in advance and bring your plan to the grocery store. Have a backup plan of healthier fast-food options and pack nutritious snacks in your car for emergencies.

# Chapter 4

1.  Macro nutrient tracking. If you are not already doing this, track your grams of protein per day for three days. Record it here:

    Day 1 _____ grams          Are you over/under? _____ grams

    Day 2 _____ grams          Are you over/under? _____ grams

    Day 3 _____ grams          Are you over/under? _____ grams

What did you find? Were you surprised?

_____

2.  Be brave! Try a new source of plant or meat protein this week. What did you try?

_____

3.  Plan ahead. Prepare a recipe with protein and vegetables as the main meal. What did you make?

_____

# Chapter 5

Make sure that *every* meal and snack includes either a fruit and/or a vegetable every day.

1.  Count your daily intake of produce for three days and record it here:

    Day 1 _____

    Day 2 _____

    Day 3 _____

2.  Try a new fruit and veggie this week. What did you try?

    New fruit: _____

    New vegetable: _____

**Examples:**

- Orange with breakfast

- Apple with mid-morning snack

- Spinach with lunch

- Broccoli and carrots with mid-day snack

- Sliced red peppers and snap peas with dinner

## Chapter 6

1. Practice reducing your number of added grams of sugar by half for the next three days and document how you feel.

_____

_____

How much more energy did you have toward the middle of day three?

_____

Do you think you could try it for a week? Yes/No

Results: _____

2. Have you ever tried sprouted or soaked grains, seeds, or legumes?

_____

Try a new sprouted grain this week and record your experience:

_____

## Chapter 7

1. How much fat are you consuming per day? Track for three days and record it here:

   Day 1 _____ grams

   Day 2 _____ grams

   Day 3 _____ grams

2. How many servings of Omega-3s are you consuming per week? _____

(Fish, flaxseed, or walnuts)

3. Exercise. Did you know that consuming added sugar in your diet without burning it off with exercise results in high triglycerides in your blood? Y/N

# Chapter 8

1.  Track your fiber intake for three days and record it here:

    Day 1 _____ grams

    Day 2 _____ grams

    Day 3 _____ grams

2.  What are some of your favorite sources of fiber?

    _____

    _____

    _____

3.  How can you get more fiber from food in your day?

    _____

    _____

4.  Do you have any additional thoughts on this subject?

    _____

    _____

    _____

# Chapter 9

1.  How much calcium are you consuming per day? Track for three days and record it here:

    Day 1 _____ servings

    Day 2 _____ servings

    Day 3 _____ servings

2.  How much vitamin D are you consuming per day? Track for three days and record it here:

    Day 1 _____ IU

    Day 2 _____ IU

    Day 3 _____ IU

3.  Practice adding one more day of strength training per week. What day will you exercise and which workout will you do?

    _____

# Chapter 10

4. If you are drinking anything with added sugar, reduce your consumption by half for three days and then get rid of it altogether for three days and document how you feel—you may feel challenged with withdrawal the first few days, so stick with it and watch your energy and immune system soar.

How did you feel when you reduced your sugar intake by half?

_____

How did you feel when you avoided added sugar in drinks for three days?

_____

5. What is one benefit of magnesium? _____

6. How much sodium do you need per day? _____

# Chapter 11

Your goal should always be to get what you need through whole foods and beverages. If you think you need a probiotic, check with your physician.  It is possible to get too much good bacteria in your stomach. If you experience bloating, gas, and diarrhea, you may have had too much sauerkraut, alcohol, or vinegar. Listen to the signs and symptoms of your body and take control of your health.

1. How does your gut feel today?

_____

Have you had any fermented foods lately?

_____

2. Try a new fermented food this week and document how you feel.

_____

# Chapter 12

What are your *new* short-term (one to six months) health goals?

_____

_____

_____

What are your *new* long-term (six months to one year) health goals?

_____

_____

How have you started overcoming the Excuse Muse?

_____

_____

Who have you discussed your goals with in the past? _____

Will you continue sharing your goals with them in the future? Yes/No

Do you believe you can become even healthier? _____ Why? _____

_____

# NOTES

## Chapter 1

Beard, Eric, Tanya Colucci, Erin McGill, and Scott Ramsdell. *NASM Live: Essentials of Personal Fitness Training*. N.p.: National Academy of Sports Medicine, 2011. Print.

Borg, Gunnar. *Borg's Perceived Exertion and Pain Scales*. Champaign, IL: Human Kinetics, 1998. Print.

Colbert, Don. *The Seven Pillars of Health*. Lake Mary, FL: Siloam, 2007. Print.

Eberle, Harold R. *Christianity Unshackled: Are You a Truth Seeker?* Shippensburg, PA: Destiny Image, 2009. Print.

Silvoso, Ed. *Anointed for Business*. Ventura, CA: Regal, 2002. Print.

TerKeurst, Lysa. *Made to Crave: Satisfying Your Deepest Desire with God, Not Food*. Grand Rapids, MI: Zondervan, 2010. Print.

## Chapter 2

Boschmann, M. "Water-Induced Thermogenesis." *Journal of Clinical Endocrinology & Metabolism* 88.12 (2003): 6015-019. Print.

"Normal Weight Ranges: Body Mass Index (BMI)." *American Cancer Society | Information and Resources for Cancer: Breast, Colon, Lung, Prostate, Skin*. American Cancer Society, 2013. Web. 19 Mar. 2013.

Clark, Micheal, Scott Lucett, and Donald T. Kirkendall. *NASM's Essentials of Sports Performance Training*. Philadelphia: Wolters Kluwer/Lippincott Williams & Wilkins, 2010. Print.

Epstein, Lawrence J., and Steven Mardon. *The Harvard Medical School Guide to a Good Night's Sleep*. New York: McGraw-Hill, 2007. Print.

"Artificial Colors." *Harvard School of Public Health*. Harvard School of Public Health, 2009. Web. 19 Mar. 2013.

Michaels, Jillian, and Mariska Van. Aalst. *Master Your Metabolism: The 3 Diet Secrets to Naturally Balancing Your Hormones for a Hot and Healthy Body!* New York: Crown, 2009. Print.

"Trans Fat Is Double Trouble for Your Heart Health." *Mayo Clinic*. Mayo Clinic, 2011. Web. 19 Mar. 2013.

"Get Enough Sleep." *United States Department of Health and Human Services*. N.p., 2013. Web. 01 Apr. 2013.

"A Food Labeling Guide: Chapter 5. Ingredients List." *US Food and Drug Administration*. N.p., 2008. Web. 10 Apr. 2013.

## Chapter 3

Clark, Micheal, Scott Lucett, and Donald T. Kirkendall. *NASM's Essentials of Sports Performance Training*. Philadelphia: Wolters Kluwer/Lippincott Williams & Wilkins, 2010. Print.

Compart, Pamela J., and Dana Godbout. Laake. *The Kid-Friendly ADHD & Autism Cookbook: The Ultimate Guide to the Gluten-Free, Casein-Free Diet*. Beverly, MA: Fair Winds, 2009. Print.

Powers, Scott K., and Edward T. Howley. *Exercise Physiology: Theory and Application to Fitness and Performance*. Boston: McGraw-Hill, 2009. Print.

Rubin, Jordan. *The Maker's Diet for Weight Loss*. Lake Mary, FL: Siloam, 2009. Print.

"Vitamin E." Dietary Supplement Fact Sheets. *Office of Dietary Supplements*, n.d. Web. 01 Apr. 2013.

## Chapter 4

Balch, Phyllis A. *Prescription for Nutritional Healing*. New York: Avery, 2000. Print.

"Center for Nutrition Policy and Promotion." *U.S. Department of Agriculture*. National Academy Press, 2010. Web. 19 Aug. 2013.

"Dietary Reference Intakes for Energy, Carbohydrate, Fiber, Fat, Fatty Acids, Cholesterol, Protein, and Amino Acids." *Food and Nutrition Board*. National Academy of Sciences, 2005. Web.

Havala, S. "Vegetarian Diets." *Journal of the American Dietetic Association* 93.11 (2003): 748-65. Print.

Powers, Scott K., and Edward T. Howley. *Exercise Physiology: Theory and Application to Fitness and Performance*. Boston: McGraw-Hill, 2009. Print.

Stokes, Tammy. *Live Your Healthiest Life: Mind, Body & Soul*. Charleston, SC: Advantage, 2010. Print.

## Chapter 5

Brennan, Georgeanne. *Salad of the Day: 365 Recipes for Every Day of the Year*. San Francisco, CA: Weldon Owen, 2012. Print.

Johnson, Duke. *The Optimal Health Revolution: How Inflammation Is the Root Cause of the Biggest Killers, How the Cutting-Edge Science of Nutrigenomics Can Transform Your Long-Term Health*. Dallas, TX: BenBella, 2009. Print.

Kidd, Kristine, and Kate Sears. *Weeknight Fresh and Fast: Simple Healthy Meals for Every Night of the Week*. San Francisco, Cal.: Weldon Owen, 2011. Print.

Stella, George. "Vegetable Stir Fry." *Food Network–Easy Recipes, Healthy Eating Ideas and Chef Recipe Videos*. N.p., n.d. Web. 01 Apr. 2013.

"Trans Fats on the Nutrition Label." U.S. Department of Agriculture. Food and Nutrition Services, n.d. Web. 19 Aug. 2013.

## Chapter 6

Ansel, Karen. "Is Gluten Bad for You." *Women's Health Magazine* Dec. 2010. N. pag. Web. 05 Apr. 2013.

Compart, Pamela J., and Dana Godbout. Laake. *The Kid-friendly ADHD & Autism Cookbook: The Ultimate Guide to the Gluten-Free, Casein-Free Diet*. Beverly, MA: Fair Winds, 2009. Print.

"Complex Carbohydrate." *The American Heritage® Dictionary of the English Language, Fifth Edition*. N.p.: Houghton Mifflin Harcourt, 2011. Print.

"Carbohydrates." *Dietary Guidelines for Americans*. United States Department of Health and Human Services, 2005. Web. 05 Apr. 2013.

Johnson, R. K., L. J. Appel, M. Brands, B. V. Howard, M. Lefevre, R. H. Lustig, F. Sacks, L. M. Steffen, and J. Wylie-Rosett. "Dietary Sugars Intake and Cardiovascular Health: A Scientific Statement From the American Heart Association." *American Heart Association* 120.11 (2009): 1011-020. Print.

Jonas, Wayne B. *Mosby's Dictionary of Complementary and Alternative Medicine*. St. Louis, MO: Mosby, 2005. Print.

"Sprouted Grain." *Food For Life*. N.p., n.d. Web. 01 Apr. 2013. http://www.foodforlife.com

## Chapter 7

Bowden, Jonny. *The 150 Healthiest Foods on Earth: The Surprising, Unbiased Truth About What You Should Eat and Why*. Gloucester, MA: Fair Winds, 2007. Print.

Compart, Pamela J., and Dana Godbout. Laake. *The Kid-friendly ADHD & Autism Cookbook: The Ultimate Guide to the Gluten-Free, Casein-Free Diet*. Beverly, MA: Fair Winds, 2009. Print.

"Dietary Reference Intakes for Energy, Carbohydrate, Fiber, Fat, Fatty Acids, Cholesterol, Protein, and Amino Acids." *Dietary Reference Intakes*. N.p., 2005. Web. 01 Apr. 2013.

Erasmus, Udo. *Fats That Heal Fats That Kill*. Burnaby, B.C.: Alive, 1993. Print.

Johnson, Duke. *The Optimal Health Revolution: How Inflammation Is the Root Cause of the Biggest Killers, How the Cutting-Edge Science of Nutrigenomics Can Transform Your Long-Term Health*. Dallas, TX: BenBella, 2009. Print.

Joseph, James A., Daniel Nadeau, and Anne Underwood. *The Color Code: A Revolutionary Eating Plan for Optimum Health*. New York: Hyperion, 2002. Print.

"Trans Fats." *Harvard School of Public Health*. Harvard School of Public Health, 2009. Web. 19 Mar. 2013.

## Chapter 8

Balch, Phyllis A. *Prescription for Nutritional Healing*. New York: Avery, 2000. Print.

"Bean Beef Burger." *Healthy Cooking* Mar. 2010: 31. Web. 05 Apr. 2013.

Johnson, Duke. *The Optimal Health Revolution: How Inflammation Is the Root Cause of the Biggest Killers, How the Cutting-Edge Science of Nutrigenomics Can Transform Your Long-Term Health*. Dallas, TX: BenBella, 2009. Print.

Krishnan, S., L. Rosenberg, M. Singer, F. B. Hu, L. Djousse, L. A. Cupples, and J. R. Palmer. "Glycemic Index, Glycemic Load, and Cereal Fiber Intake and Risk of Type 2 Diabetes in US Black Women." *Archives of Internal Medicine* 167.21 (2007): 2304-309. Print.

Mellen, P., T. Walsh, and D. Herrington. "Whole Grain Intake and Cardiovascular Disease: A Meta-analysis." *Nutrition, Metabolism and Cardiovascular Diseases* 18.4 (2008): 283-90. Print.

Pereira, M. "Dietary Fiber and Risk of Coronary Heart Disease." *ACC Current Journal Review* 13.5 (2004): 26. Print.

## Chapter 9

"Are You at Risk?" *National Osteoporosis Foundation*. N.p., n.d. Web. 05 Apr. 2013.

Balch, Phyllis A. *Prescription for Nutritional Healing*. New York: Avery, 2000. Print.

Bloom, Sophie. "What Are the Dangers of Synthetic Vitamins?" *LIVESTRONG.COM*. N.p., 13 July 2010. Web. 05 Apr. 2013.

Holick, MF. "Sunlight and Vitamin D for Bone Health and Prevention of Autoimmune Diseases, Cancers, and Cardiovascular Disease." *American Journal of Clinical Nutrition* 88S Dec.167S (2004): 80. Print.

Johnson, Duke. *The Optimal Health Revolution: How Inflammation Is the Root Cause of the Biggest Killers, How the Cutting-Edge Science of Nutrigenomics Can Transform Your Long-Term Health*. Dallas, TX: BenBella, 2009. Print.

Staff, Mayo Clinic. "Dietary Fiber: Essential for a Healthy Diet." *Mayo Clinic*. Mayo Foundation for Medical Education and Research, 17 Nov. 2012. Web. 19 Mar. 2013.

"What Is Osteoarthritis?" *United States Department of Health and Human Services | HHS.gov*. National Institute of Arthritis and Musculoskeletal and Skin Diseases, Nov. 2010. Web. 19 Aug. 2013.

## Chapter 10

Abdelkafi, Sofia. "8 Homemade Vitamin Water Recipes." *Sofia Abdelkafi Registred Dietitian*. N.p., n.d. Web. 12 Apr. 2013.

Bowden, Jonny. *The Most Effective Natural Cures on Earth: The Surprising, Unbiased Truth about What Treatments Work and Why*. Beverly, MA: Fair Winds, 2008. Print.

Carlos, Juan. "Scientists Link Excess Sugar to Cancer." *Medical Research Journal* Feb (2013): n. pag. Print.

Compart, Pamela J., and Dana Godbout Laake. *The Kid-friendly ADHD & Autism Cookbook: The Ultimate Guide to the Gluten-Free, Casein-Free Diet*. Beverly, MA: Fair Winds, 2009. Print.

"Dietary Guidelines for Americans." Health.gov. US Department of Health and Human Services, n.d. Web. 05 Apr. 2013.

Johnson, R. K., L. J. Appel, M. Brands, B. V. Howard, M. Lefevre, R. H. Lustig, F. Sacks, L. M. Steffen, and J. Wylie-Rosett. "Dietary Sugars Intake and Cardiovascular Health: A Scientific Statement From the American Heart Association." *Circulation* 120.11 (2009): 1011-020. Print.

"Just Give Me the FACTS!" *Cereal FACTS–Home*. Yale University, 2009. Web. 12 Apr. 2013.

McMillen, S. I. *None of These Diseases*. [Westwood, N.J.]: F. H. Revell, 2000. Print.

Michaels, Jillian, and Mariska Van Aalst. *Master Your Metabolism: The 3 Diet Secrets to Naturally Balancing Your Hormones for a Hot and Healthy Body!* New York: Crown, 2009. Print.

Queen's University. "Chemists Shed Light on Health Benefits of Garlic." *Science Daily* Jan (2009): n. pag. Print.

"Release 25." *Nutrient Data Products and Services*. N.p., n.d. Web. 12 Apr. 2013.

"Shaking the Salt Habit." *American Heart Association*, 22 Apr. 2013. Web. 05 May 2013.

Skorecki K, Ausiello D. *Disorders of Sodium and Water Homeostasis*, In: Goldman L, Schafer AI, eds. *Goldman's Cecil Medicine*, 24th ed. Philadelphia, Pa.: Elsevier Saunders; 2011: chap 118.

"Sodium and Chloride." *Dietary Reference Intakes*. USDA Food and Nutrition Information, n.d. Web. 01 Apr. 2013.

Staff, Mayo Clinic. "Added Sugar: Don't Get Sabotaged by Sweeteners." *Mayo Clinic*. Mayo Foundation for Medical Education and Research, 05 Oct. 2012. Web. 05 Apr. 2013.

TerKeurst, Lysa. *Made to Crave: Satisfying Your Deepest Desire with God, Not Food*. Grand Rapids, MI: Zondervan, 2010. Print.

## Chapter 11

Balch, Phyllis A. *Prescription for Nutritional Healing*. New York: Avery, 2000. Print.

Costenbader, Carol W. *The Big Book of Preserving the Harvest*. North Adams, MA: Storey, 2002. Print.

Katz, Sandor. "Making Sauerkraut." *Wild Fermentation*. N.p., 27 Apr. 2012. Web. 19 Apr. 2013.

Katz, Sandor Ellix. *Wild Fermentation: The Flavor, Nutrition, and Craft of Live-culture Foods*. White River Junction, VT: Chelsea Green Pub., 2003. Print.

McMillen, S. I. *None of These Diseases*. [Westwood, N.J.]: F. H. Revell, 2000. Print.

Seidenberg, Casey. "Fermented Foods Bubble with Healthful Benefits." *Washington Post*. The Washington Post, 20 Nov. 2012. Web. 19 Apr. 2013.

## Chapter 12

Batterson, Mark. *The Circle Maker: Praying Circles around Your Biggest Dreams and Greatest Fears*. Grand Rapids, MI: Zondervan, 2011. Print.

Dunbar, Brian. "Frequently Asked Questions." *NASA*. Kennedy Space Center, 01 May 2013. Web. 19 Apr. 2013.

# ACKNOWLEDGMENTS

God is holy. I am at peace. Thank you God for the gift of voice and relationship.

First and foremost, thank you to my husband, Casey, for his unwavering confidence, patience, strength, and encouragement in everything I do. My beautiful little children Isabella and Kane who keep me on my tippy toes, giggling with them all day long.

My family: Debra, Tony, Dave, Rosie, John, and Tony for their support and love; my three sisters Sara, Caitlyn, and Alexis, who hold fragrant petals of tenderness in my heart; Ryan, Brent, Lisa, Tracy, Billie, and Aaron, in whose incredible families I am an addition and who helped shape my life growing up.

My dear, beloved friends for believing in me, helping me, and keeping me balanced.

Colleagues for their encouragement and insight.

Clients for being my true inspiration for this book.

Contributor and honest friend Christina Zaczkowski, who helped to paint the pages of the affirmations with rich color and vibrant depth; Bjorn Dixon for his admirable foreword, which offers hope for health that reaches far beyond the physical body.

Business affiliates who walk along side my mission for a healthier community.

Editors: Specifically my cherished aunt Catherine Long for her careful and detailed work, patience, and teaching; Hanna Kjeldbjerg and the whole team at Beaver's Pond Press for their expertise; my adored friend and mentor Tracy Shearer; loyal directors, assistants, advisors, and friends Carmen Trainor, Shannon Immer, Tracy and Rob Rowe, Kim Hanauska, James Zaczkowski, Stephanie Klinzing, Trudy Webb, Steve Fessler, and Mike Schoemer. This book would not be possible without you; to my corporate promotions professional Julie Frandsen; and designers Alicia Black and Jay Monroe to see things I could never see.

Photography by Jacki Vaughan, owner of jacki v. photography, and cosmetologist, Aarica Larson, owner of InSPAration Salon.

And last but certainly not least, you, my readers, who I may not meet in person but who invest in themselves through this book, to seek something *unique*—you are worth *more than mediocre, you are worth being the best you can be*. Thank you for entrusting me with your health. I pray this book would be a blessing as you live in wellness.

# INDEX

# ABOUT ASHLEY

**A**shley Darkenwald, BA, CPT, PES, has been a professional in the fitness industry for over a decade. Her passion for health and fitness started as a gymnastics athlete and then coach. Years ago, one of her first fitness commitments was to exercise every day for just three minutes, and now she has become a nationally-accredited certified personal trainer, fitness instructor, speaker, mother of two, President of InFIT, and an Anytime Fitness Franchise owner. Ashley is a motivational powerhouse and is excited for you to join her on an amazing and positive journey toward optimal health and fitness.

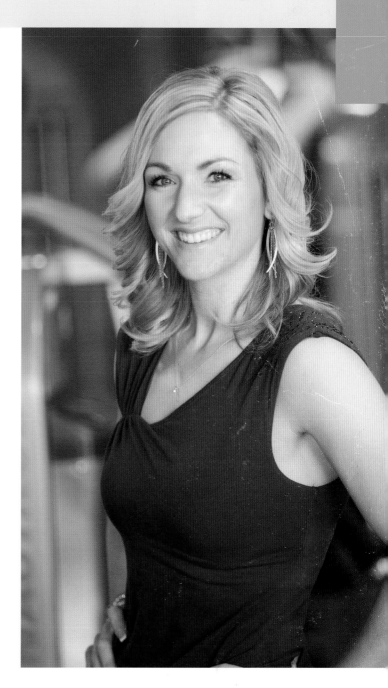